ETHICS

CONFLICTS OF INTEREST

ETHICS

CONFLICTS OF INTEREST

Edited by

Verena Tschudin BSc (Hons), RGN, RM,
Dip. Counselling

Illustrations by Richard Smith

Scutari Press · London

A division of Scutari Projects Ltd, the publishing company of the Royal College of Nursing

First published 1994

British Library Cataloguing in Publication Data
Conflicts of Interest. – (Ethics Series)
  I. Tschudin, Verena II. Series
  170
    ISBN 1–873853–10–6

Phototypeset by Intype, London
Printed by Bell and Bain Ltd., Glasgow

Contents

Contributors

Maureen Eby BA, AASc, FETC, PGDip, RN

Lecturer in Medical and Surgical Nursing, University of Birmingham

Bob Gates MSc, BEd(Hons), DipN(Lond), RNMH, RMN, CertEd, RNT

Lecturer in Nursing, University of Hull

Ann Leedham MA, BA(Hons), RGN, RNT, DipN(Lond)

Full-time Officer, Royal College of Nursing

Preface

Ethics is not only at the heart of nursing, it *is* the heart of nursing. Ethics is about what is right and good. Nursing and caring are synonymous, and the way in which care is carried out is ethically decisive. How a patient is addressed, cared for and treated must be right not only by ordinary standards of care, but also by ethical principles.

These ethical principles have not always been addressed clearly, but now patients, nurses, doctors and all types of health care personnel are questioning their care in the light of ethics. Their starting points and approaches are different, but their 'results' are remarkably similar. The individual person matters and the care given and received has to be human and humanising.

The way in which the contributors to this volume, and others in the series, address their subject is also individual and unique. Their brief was simply that what they wrote should be applicable to practising nurses. Each chapter reflects the personal style and approach of the writer. This is what gives this series its distinctive character and strength, and provides the reader with the opportunity to see different approaches working. It is hoped that this will encourage readers to think that their own way of understanding ethics and behaving ethically is also acceptable and worthwhile. Theories and principles are important, and so are their interpretation and application. That is a job for everybody, not just the experts: experts can point the way – as in this series of books — but all nurses need to be challenged and encouraged.

Emphasis is laid in all the chapters on the individual nurse and patient or client. Ethics 'happens' between and among people, and, by the authors bringing their own experience to bear on their chapters, they show how ethics works in relationships.

Great achievements often start with a small idea quite different from the end result, and so it is with this series of books. The initial proposal is almost unrecognisable in the final product. Many people contributed to the growth of the idea, many more were involved in implementing it, and I hope that even more will benefit from it.

My particular thanks go to Geoff Hunt, Director of the European Centre for Professional Ethics, for his advice and help with this series.

Verena Tschudin

CHAPTER 1

Refusal to Care

Bob Gates

With an increasing awareness of personal and professional
values has also gone an increasing awareness of the possible
conflict between them. Personal and professional rights and
responsibilities are not always clear; an ethic of caring can be
seen as a basis on which to judge and decide.

   This chapter highlights some of the reasons why refusal to
give care to a patient might be considered and carried out. The
author outlines the basic difficulties using case studies as
examples, thus helping the reader to see the wider
implications of caring and being cared for.

What Is Meant by Refusal to Care

The first part of this chapter attempts to articulate an
operational definition of what we understand and therefore
mean by the term 'refusal to care'. In addition, the concept
and practice of caring is explored. The remaining parts of
the chapter will then explore the background discussion
of refusal to care, followed by examples and short case
histories.

   The chapter is couched in the ideology of caring and
attempts to encourage readers to understand refusal to care
as a complex ethical dilemma. This will be explored from
a number of different perspectives.

   Refusal to care within this chapter means:

   A conscious decision by a nurse practitioner to refuse to
   meet the needs of a patient in her or his nursing
   interventions. These needs are global and include the

physical, psychological, social, intellectual and spiritual dimensions of human existence. Refusal relates to a knowing and conscious decision, because it implies that the practitioner is able to choose between providing or refusing nursing care.

The caring relationship

The relationship between caring and ethics in nursing has been well explored by Tschudin (1986). Caring is portrayed as the nurse — a human being — in a relationship with another human being. In such a relationship there is respect for the other person, and this leads to clarity of the relationship. In addition, such a relationship enables the other person to express himself or herself freely and allows the nurse to empathise, while retaining a separateness in order not to be overwhelmed by the relationship. Lastly, the relationship should help the other person to grow and develop, aided by the nurse communicating support for this person.

In a sense, the promotion of caring in our relationships with people is a renaissance of the fundamental nature of nursing. It stems from a deep and profound concern for humanity which transcends contracts and the current ideology of the 'marketplace' within health care. Given the characteristics of a caring relationship, conscious voluntary actions by nurses which violate or compromise the caring characteristics should be seen as a refusal to care for a person.

Conscious or unconscious refusal

Based on the writings of Aristotle, Thompson, Melia and Boyd (1988) point out that one cannot be held responsible for actions carried out involuntarily or in ignorance. Thus, refusal to care must be conscious or voluntary to be prob-

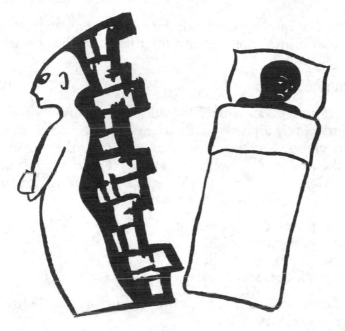

lematic. A conscious decision may be motivated by a variety of factors and applied either overtly or covertly to patients being cared for. However, the issue of who defines both need and care is problematic. If care is defined solely from a medical perspective, any nurse not wishing to be associated with this care is immediately labelled as someone refusing to care for that patient.

The nurse–doctor relationship

The nature of the relationship between doctor and nurse has been written about by many people. There is an excellent account of the complexities of this relationship in Brown, Kitson and McKnight (1992). They ascribe most of the existing problems to tradition, hierarchy and failure to communicate well between the professions. These authors claim that, if there is to be more flexibility in professional roles and more team work, and if increasing medical and nursing demands are to be met, patients need to assume more responsibility for their own healthcare.

Rights and duties

Burnard and Chapman (1988) discuss the issue of rights and duty. They argue that a patient may be said to possess certain rights, and, as a corollary of this, the nurse has incumbent duties. The International Council of Nurses (ICN) *Code for Nurses* (1973) specifies four major areas related to a nurse's duties. These are:

- the promotion of health;
- the prevention of illness;
- the restoration of health;
- the alleviation of suffering.

Such duties are an integral component of any discussion concerning ethics.

Ethical frameworks

Marr (1992) provides a useful summary of two classical theoretical perspectives of ethics. No apology is made here for briefly outlining them, because it is these two perspectives that will be used as the basis for discussion within this chapter.

The first, **utilitarianism** (generically referred to as consequentialism), is concerned with acts which enable the greatest good for the greatest number of people.

The second theoretical approach explored here is that of **deontology** (generically known as non-consequentialism). This asserts the duty to arrive at actions which are good in themselves, regardless of the consequences.

Utilitarianism promotes the greatest good for the greatest number, acknowledging and understanding conse-

quences of actions and conforming to rules which promote
these ideals. The second approach, deontology, concentrates upon the here-and-now resolution of dilemmas and
goodness for its own sake, regardless of the consequences.

As with all theoretical approaches, utilitarianism and
deontology provide us with a framework of reference to
use, both in reading about them and when practising
nursing. Seldom, however, can such theoretical approaches
be applied to the multiplicity of contexts in which we as
practitioners work. In order to do this, we need to be able
to analyse and synthesise theory and formulate this into
reflective practice. Tschudin (1992) acknowledges the difficulty of following a single theoretical approach when she
says:

> It seems difficult to act without thinking of the
> consequences at all, or to act thinking only of the
> consequences.

Such a stance prompts Ellis (1993) to argue for a com-
bined view of theoretical perspectives:

> The most satisfactory way of resolving ethical dilemmas is
> to combine the best features of both utility and deontology
> . . . Applying this sort of combined view of ethics enables
> professionals to act within the confines of their code of
> conduct and take account of their own beliefs and cultural/
> sociological influences as well as those of their clients.

Let us now move on to tease out, as it were, the background discussion to the issues surrounding refusal to care.

Refusal to Care: Some Examples

Within this section examples of refusal to care from the
literature are woven together with the theoretical perspectives of ethics already outlined.

Thompson, Melia and Boyd (1988) provide an example of a man aged 27 with hepatitis and renal failure. He was on dialysis and was progressing, although not as well as expected. The consultant involved in the care of this man decided that the dialysis machine could be put to better use on other patients, so the man was taken off the machine and prescribed diamorphine. A number of nurses refused to administer this medication, because of his age and prognosis. Clearly the nurses were refusing to care for this patient — or were they? Who defines care and treatment?

It may be that the personnel involved in this example were approaching the dilemma from different theoretical perspectives. The consultant might be said to be making ethical decisions within the utilitarianist perspective, that is, considering the greatest good for the greatest number. The nurses could be said to be making decisions within the deontological perspective, that is, the pursuance of their ethical duty to act correctly, regardless of the consequences, vis-à-vis their patient. In a study on ethical decision-making processes by doctors and nurses, Grundstein (1992) suggests that the two professions act out different values and expectations. Nurses would appear to place a greater emphasis on a caring perspective. Doctors, on the other hand, place an emphasis on patients' rights. Such a finding supports the need to understand refusal to care from a number of different perspectives.

Refusing to care by not participating in the administration of electroconvulsive therapy (ECT) was an extremely sensitive topic a few years ago. St Augustine's Hospital in Canterbury, Kent, acknowledged that a degree of force had been used to administer ECT to unwilling and informal patients (Beardshaw, 1981). Clearly and paradoxically, a nurse would have an ethical duty to refuse to be involved in such a care regime. However, refusing to care is potentially damaging to nurses, even if those nurses have a strong ethical base guiding their actions.

Another example of refusal to care is that of a senior nursing officer at Wrexham Park Hospital who refused to comply with medical colleagues' wishes in a number of areas related to both medical and nursing care (Walsh 1982). Walsh complained that information was falsified and that treatment was forcibly administered. His eventual suspension was brought about by his refusal to instruct staff to hold down a patient while a tranquilliser was administered, because he felt that such an act was a violation of the Mental Health Act (1959).

The issue of refusing to care for someone because a nurse perceives him or her as an unlikeable person is another area to consider. An important contribution to understanding in this area is offered by Stockwell (1984). From her study, Stockwell concluded that some nurses enjoyed caring for some patients more than others. Unpopularity of patients, in her study, appeared to be related to personality factors, physical defects and ethnic origin. Nurses gave least attention to bedfast patients who were neither overtly popular nor unpopular.

Stockwell's study is fundamentally important if we are to understand the possible reasons why nurses may decide to refuse to care for a patient. Such a decision can be based upon something as relatively straightforward and yet as complex as the nature of social interaction. This is of great significance, for if a nurse is unable to care for a patient because of a dislike of the patient, and therefore consciously refuses to care, how is she or he able to promote health, restore health or alleviate suffering, as is required by the ICN *Code for Nurses* (1973)? Brown, Kitson and McKnight (1992) raise this issue when they ask:

> what happens if we find that we cannot care for a particular patient, when our personal reaction is one of distrust,

repugnance or hate? Is it acceptable to admit that there will
be some people for whom we as human beings cannot
care?

Another area in which nurses have refused to care concerns people with human immunodeficiency virus (HIV)
and acquired immune deficiency syndrome (AIDS).
Huerta and Oddi (1992) suggest that, historically, nurses
have accepted the risk of contagion while caring for people
with an infectious disease. However, coupled with the
concerns of contagion go other factors such as fear, ignorance and homophobia. These additional factors may
influence a nurse's decision in refusing to care for such a
client (Huerta and Oddi, 1992). Sim (1992) examines this
issue and suggests that in relation to nursing patients with
HIV or AIDS, nurses undertake a process of risk assessment. In this process, nurses may feel that risk is raised to
an unacceptable threshold, which may then lead them
to 'abrogate the usual duty to treat'. Sim (1992), in argument against such an abrogation of duty, concludes that:

> it is inconsistent with normal professional practice, and with
> the underlying professional ethic of nursing, to argue for
> a no-risk position. By its very nature, health care carries
> some degree of risk, and nurses who are unwilling to
> accept this have misunderstood the nature of their
> professional role.

A Typology of Refusal to Care

Refusal to care has thus been shown to manifest itself in
a variety of types of human behaviour (Figure 1).

At least four main types of refusal to care can be demon-
strated. These are based upon prejudice, competing ethical
demands, professional negligence and interpersonal skills
failure.

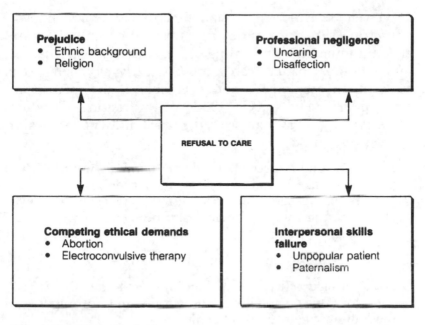

Fig. 1 Typology of refusal to care

Although the typologies are depicted as separate entities, it should be remembered that they are constructs or reflections of reality, so are not mutually exclusive. Prejudice, for example, may result in interpersonal skills failure, and vice versa.

The typology is embryonic and has only been developed to give some structure to the way in which we understand refusal to care. Readers should be able further to explore and develop this typology based upon their own practice as nurses.

Prejudice

It is a regrettable but haunting reality that prejudice is to be found in most communities, of which nursing is no exception. Prejudice based upon ethnic origin and religion may well be experienced and practised by some nurses. Sampson (1982) points out that hospital communities are not immune from the strong feelings that racial, cultural and religious matters can arouse. Clearly any behaviour based upon prejudice is not acceptable in any form from nursing staff. The UKCC Code of Professional Conduct (1992) says that as a registered nurse, midwife or health visitor, one must:

> Recognise and respect the uniqueness and dignity of each patient and client, and respond to their need for care, irrespective of their ethnic origin, religious beliefs, personal attributes, the nature of their health problems or any other factor.

However, Tak Leung Chan (1993) says:

> None of us is actually neutral and nurses should always be aware of their own cultural expectations and not impose these upon clients from different cultures.

This is an important observation, because if we attempt to adopt a caring position in our nursing actions, we may well find a conflict in our inner values between the central tenets of caring and the 'ghosts' of our own cultural experience. Therefore, the Royal College of Nursing (1976) has advised its members that:

> Discrimination against particular individuals, for whatever reason, should never be tolerated . . . The adoption of a professional attitude requires that all those who need nursing care should receive it without discrimination.

In a sense, the UKCC Code of Professional Conduct (1992) is superfluous in this area, as there are no moral or ethical precedents which would support prejudice within an ideology of human caring. However, prejudice *is* present, and nurses may well find themselves experiencing strong emotional feelings towards people for whom they are expected to care. It is important for practitioners to bring to the surface, as it were, their feelings toward people of a different colour, ethnic origin, religion or class. Can *your* feelings lead you to act in a prejudicial manner? If you hold prejudices, do you wish to pursue the ideology of caring and explore ways in which you can develop positive images of people from backgrounds different from your own?

Competing ethical demands

Utilitarianism (consequentialism) exists to pursue the greatest good for the greatest number. By contrast, deontology (non-consequentialism) seeks to promote that which is right regardless of the outcome. This may lead to a nurse experiencing competing ethical demands. Such a situation may be characterised by a nurse engaging in actions based upon a theoretical framework which, paradoxically, may manifest itself as appearing unethical. An example of this may be that of a nurse refusing to care for a woman having a termination of pregnancy. Refusing to participate in aspects of termination of pregnancy may be seen as ethically justified if the decision to refuse to care is based upon a higher moral or ethical principle than merely refusing to care. Such issues of conscience are explored by Rumbold (1986) and also include such areas as ECT, amniocentesis and unnecessary treatment.

Professional negligence

Within this type of refusal to care are examples of uncaring behaviour and disaffection. For a nurse to act in an uncaring manner is, in a sense, a refusal to care. To choose to deny care to a patient is perhaps a conscious attempt to refuse to give something to which human beings in need of nursing care are entitled.

Disaffection refers to individual nurses who have become alienated or disconnected from the value systems of the organisation for which they work or from the profession of nursing as a whole. This may result in nurses consciously refusing to care for patients because the central tenets of the caring philosophy are no longer present.

Nurses who become disaffected or uncaring may be charged with professional negligence (Beardshaw, 1981).

Interpersonal skills failure

This last type of refusal to care is based upon the failure, at an interpersonal level, of nurses and patients to share congruent, effective communication, and upon a failure to develop a trusting relationship based on the principles of caring. Such failure may be traced to the patient being perceived as unpopular. Alternatively, the nurse may adopt a parentalistic approach to caring for people.

In relation to a patient being unpopular, Thompson, Melia and Boyd (1988) say:

> Unpopular patients may . . . be at some risk of having their psychological if not physical needs undervalued.

Parentalism is sometimes manifest in nurses refusing to care because the person being cared for is perceived as 'having brought it upon himself' ('it' being the current condition). While this may not lead to a total denial of care, such 'parental' comments are nevertheless sometimes overtly expressed by carers. An example may be the young man or woman in an Accident and Emergency department who has taken an overdose. It is not uncommon to find practitioners saying that they are wasting their time, or that the patients are just seeking attention and so on. Napier (1985) says, concerning AIDS:

> frankly I have no sympathy with homosexuals who contract

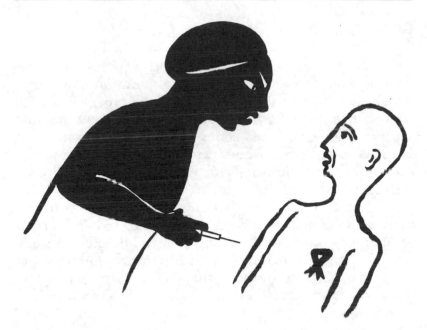

the disease. This is because it has been contracted through performing an unnatural act: a biological fact. Therefore, while nurses have a duty to care for the sick, we must also recognise that it is 'self inflicted' in the truest sense of the term, and need not have arisen in the first place. What makes AIDS more horrific is that a stranger's perverse sexual actions can harm totally unknown innocents.

Parentalism may also be evident when nurses do not tell the truth. If the other person in the caring relationship is not told the truth, how can the relationship be said to be caring? Is the nurse consciously choosing not to adopt the ideology of caring and all that such an ideology requires? Are you always able to communicate freely and openly with the person for whom you care? In relation to with-holding truth, Martin (1993) says:

the active participation of patients in their own treatment should be facilitated by means of open, sensitive, and honest communication.

Case Histories of Refusal to Care

Figure 1 (above) identified four types of refusal to care. This section of the chapter portrays four case histories which demonstrate characteristics of the types described. The case histories are authentic and represent real-life nursing situations. The names and locations of the case histories have been changed to protect the anonymity of those involved. The details of the actions which followed the scenarios are not presented.

This particular section is designed to engage you in a process of 'armchair' reflection exercises. It is important for us as practitioners of nursing to spend time in critically reflecting on and analysing our nursing care. Therefore, at the end of the case histories there are a number of questions which you might consider answering for yourself.

Kenny

Kenny was a 32-year-old man with profound learning disabilities, living on a ward in a large hospital caring for people with learning disabilities. Each ward within the hospital essentially catered for a particular dependency group, his particular ward being for people with challenging behaviours.

Kenny was a good-looking man with a winning smile. Unfortunately, while living at the hospital, he acquired a number of behaviours which were seen as problematic. Kenny would, if not directly observed, snatch and bolt food in vast quantities. On one occasion, he managed to consume practically the whole supper for all the men on the ward. He would frequently become incontinent, both of urine and faeces, despite being toileted every two hours or so.

Kenny also had the ability singlehandedly to annoy all the men on the ward at the same time. When in the mood, he would slowly move around the ward either hitting or pinching each of the men, one at a time, until they became agitated.

After approximately half an hour, all the men on the ward would start to show exaggerated challenging behaviours. Consequently, Kenny was disliked by the majority of the nursing staff on the ward. The two charge nurses noted that if a group was organised to go swimming, for a walk or for some social outing, Kenny was always excluded. If extra food or snacks were available, Kenny was overlooked. In general, nurses would consciously avoid offering Kenny the same levels or opportunities of care as they offered the other men on the ward.

Kenny was essentially an unliked man, and because of this, nurses would consciously refuse aspects of nursing care to him, even if they found difficulty in articulating that this was what they were doing. The two charge nurses became increasingly worried about the ethical implications of such actions by their nursing colleagues.

Julia and Robert

This case history was related by a senior nurse in charge of a unit for children with a learning disability and superimposed physical and/or sensory handicap. The events took place in a London borough during the 1980s. The children were profoundly disabled, both in terms of their ability to learn and in the degree and extent of their physical disability. The unit was located in a multicultural community, where ethnic tensions were a common experience of everyday life.

The unit was divided into three 'homes', each of which was an integral part of a larger building. Each home had its own staffing establishment, although during periods of sickness or absenteeism, staff would be moved to another area to make the best use of the resources. The senior nurse would also cover the areas himself when circumstances required him to do so. It was during one such period when the senior nurse was covering for a member of staff on 'blue' house that the following incident took place.

The staff on duty on the morning of the incident were the senior nurse, an enrolled nurse (learning disability) and a care

assistant (learning disability). The enrolled nurse was a black
nurse and the care assistant was a white nurse. In common
with many 'ordinary' homes, a pattern emerged in the caring
practices of the care staff, where first thing in the morning the
children were woken, washed, dressed and breakfasted.
Because of the profound disabilities of the children, the senior
nurse assumed that the nursing staff helped one another with
those children who were the most dependent. Julia and Robert,
both profoundly disabled, and white, really needed two nurses
to help them. It soon emerged that the enrolled nurse would not
help with the dressing of the white children and the care
assistant would not help with the black children. At this time,
the enrolled nurse was caring for one of the less dependent
black children. The senior nurse overheard a series of sarcastic
and racist comments between the two nurses. After talking to
both nurses at some length, it emerged that nurses in all three
of the 'homes' frequently refused to care for children if they
were of an ethnic origin different from themselves. The senior
nurse was both devastated and disgusted. He immediately
moved the care assistant and provided oral warnings (pending
further investigations) of discipline to both the care assistant
and the enrolled nurse.

Raymond

This case history is concerned with a young man who lived by
himself in a rather run-down bedsit on the outskirts of a large
town. He presented himself to the Accident and Emergency
department of his local hospital complaining of prolonged and
severe abdominal pain for the last two days. Following his
medical examination, the house officer diagnosed acute
appendicitis which warranted an emergency appendectomy,
and Raymond was transferred to the surgical ward.

When he arrived on the ward, one could not but notice his
appearance. He was shabby, untidy and obviously had not
bathed or washed for several days. He smelt of both body odour
and urine. His fingernails were long, and there was a thick

black line of matter embedded under them. His hair was long, and his scalp was encrusted with dandruff. Clearly, Raymond needed a bath to prepare him for his surgery.

A staff nurse and a student nurse were asked by the ward sister to ensure that he was bathed and made ready for theatre. After the ward sister had left, the staff nurse asked if she could discuss something with the student nurse outside the bay area where Raymond was. When they were both in a quiet area, the staff nurse explained that Raymond made her feel physically sick. She went on to explain to the student nurse that she would have to bathe Raymond by herself. She said that she would explain the situation to the ward sister who she knew would understand. The student nurse replied that she did understand the staff nurse's difficulties but that they should not cause her to refuse to care for Raymond. Following a heated discussion, the student nurse left to go and bathe Raymond by herself.

Michael

A staff nurse on an acute admission ward for people with mental health problems remembers the following story which took place in 1978, and which is reported in his own words.

'It was my privilege to spend some time caring for Michael. He was an intensely private man in his late 50s. He had a history of agitated depression, resulting in repeated voluntary admission to his local psychiatric hospital. He was a draughtsman by trade and, according to his wife and friends, was very good at his job. On his admission, he was extremely depressed and agitated. He was tearful and spent long periods wringing his hands and repeatedly saying, "I am no good for anyone, I always let everybody down."

'Because of the loving care of his wife, he was never unkempt on admission and she always managed to get him to drink plenty, even though he often went for long periods when he did not bother to eat. I spent most of the day of his admission reassuring him and encouraging him to relax.

'Multidisciplinary team meetings were commonly used to discuss newly admitted patients in order to agree a treatment regime. At the meeting when Michael's care was being discussed, the consultant psychiatrist admitted to being "foxed" as to knowing what to do next. All attempts at controlling Michael's depression had failed to bring about any long-lasting benefit. Eventually, the psychiatrist concluded that only one avenue remained unexplored: the use of ECT. This idea was met with instant reservations by the charge nurse of the ward. He articulated the opinion that the use of ECT was seldom more effective than the use of antidepressant medication. The discussion between the charge nurse and the consultant was tense, and it was agreed that it should be continued after the meeting. However, it was agreed at the meeting that Michael would be offered the option of ECT as a treatment. It was further agreed that this should be discussed with Michael and his wife as soon as possible.

'After the meeting, I spoke with the charge nurse, who was clearly very angry. He was incensed with the arrogance of the consultant; he complained, "What is the point of team meetings when one person effectively makes all the decisions?" I attempted to calm the charge nurse, saying that it was really up to Michael and his wife to decide which was the best form of treatment. At this point, the consultant entered the office to finish the "discussion". Without waiting for the consultant to speak, the charge nurse said, "I think it is morally wrong to give Michael ECT . . . he is in no position to make an informed choice; if you go ahead with this I refuse to have anything to do with it. Someone else will have to care for him because I think it is unethical." '

Reflecting on the case studies

You might like to spend some time now reflecting on these case histories.

- Try to identify which type of refusal to care each

case history represents and which particular category it might fall into.

- Why and how do you think situations such as these can occur?
- How do you think you might respond to the ethical dilemmas posed, should you ever find yourself in a similar situation?
- How do you usually resolve ethical dilemmas in your practice?
- What, in your experience, makes an ethical decision-making process useful? (Chapter 4 may be helpful here.)

You may want to discuss some of these issues with friends or colleagues.

Implications and Discussion

The purpose of this last section of this chapter is to bring together the points made thus far and to discuss the implications of refusal to care.

Given the dimensions of caring, can a nurse refuse to care? Sim (1992) says:

> any policy of avoidance or refusal to treat must be thought through to its logical consequences, and should not be considered solely in terms of a one-to-one nurse–patient relationship.

Reflect on a possible scenario when you, as a practitioner, might choose to refuse to care for a person. What would the outcome of such a decision be? Is it possible that if you refuse to care, other nurse practitioners may also refuse to care? An obvious consequence of one nurse's refusal to care may be collective refusal to care. Stated simply, the patient will not be cared for.

As a practitioner of nursing you must ask yourself whether this could ever be ethically justified. There is a need to deliberate in areas of potential ethical dilemmas, and the issue of refusal to care must be seen as an area where such deliberation is required in any resolution of problems. Brown, Kitson and McKnight (1992) outline the stages of deliberation which occur in relation to ethical dilemmas.

1. Appreciation of the situation and possible outcomes.
2. Review of possible courses of action.
3. Selection and application of principles.
4. Weighing of practical considerations.
5. Decision-making.

Stage 1 requires a practitioner to identify and prioritise the elements of the situation into (a) important features and (b) features which could be thought of as marginal. Stage 2 requires a mapping out of various courses of action which could be pursued. In Stage 3, the practitioner must consider the dilemma against personal principles which originate from past experience, one's values of caring and the nurse's professional Code of Conduct. These principles will lead the practitioner to consider a particular course of action. In Stage 4, the practitioner is required to consider her or his proposed response in the light of the current working context and the consequences which may follow. Stage 5 is the decision-making stage. A clearly-defined process of deliberation helps to reach a resolution and response to the dilemma which is thought out rather than being a reflex response.

In a sense, we are all in a position to be able to refuse to care for people. However, such a decision is likely to affect us as practitioners, as well as the person being cared for. Brown, Kitson and McKnight (1992) suggest that this will manifest itself at the 'natural and ethical' levels.

Concerning the natural level, they make the statement that:

> If we did not want to care and be cared for, if we did not mind suffering and were not liable to despair or if such experiences could not be helped by companionship, then we would not need to put such a high value on caring.

This natural level of caring enables the nurse practitioner to develop an ethic of caring. At the ethical level, they suggest that:

> The basic notions about caring come from our own biographies, our experiences of being cared for. These supply a form that can be recognised as caring impulses. . . To be the person one wants to be in relation to the wellbeing of others and to facilitate their good before one's own is a clear declaration of one's ethical position.

In other words, to adopt a subjective mode of caring, as opposed to a more objective and distancing form of nursing, requires the nurse to give of her or himself in the truest sense. This giving inevitably extends beyond the fixed requirements of professional codes and contracts. Because of this, caring is given at a personal cost to the nurse practitioner.

It can also be argued that caring has been professionalised, or in a sense institutionalised, by the nursing profession. What is purported as caring may be no more than a convenient display of concern, with little or no depth to the relationship. There is a substantive difference between the professional nature of caring given by nurses and the caring that is found in true and deeply personal social relationships. Brown, Kitson and McKnight (1992) discuss this issue at length, making a distinction between lay and professional values.

Melia (1987) also points out these differences. Firstly, she says, nursing is a paid and contracted service between an employer and an employee (the nurse). Secondly, nurses are not involved in the other person's life on an individual basis as are friends and/or family. Lastly, there is an incongruity between the nurse's values, lifestyle and culture and that of the person whom she or he is nursing.

Given these potential differences, is it right to expect that a nurse should be able to care for a person in the way in which the ideology of caring is promoted? A range of points raised in defence of both positions needs to be considered, and values of both need to be seen, before conclusions are drawn whether or not caring, in the way described, is an attainable reality for practitioners of nursing.

It is appropriate, therefore, briefly to revisit the issue of who defines care in the context of the nurse– or doctor–patient relationship, which was earlier identified as, in some instances, problematic. Perhaps we need to move beyond our historical rhetoric of 'mud slinging' with our medical colleagues. The person most central to the debate in such dilemmas is the 'other person' in the caring relationship. If control of decision-making needs a fixed location, people must be empowered to assume their own responsibility. This said, nurses and doctors do need to respect each other's professional position in the caring relationship. Walsh (1982), quoted earlier, said:

> The consultants have tried to determine what nursing care is — and we have denied them that.

Nurses cannot and should not attempt to work in isolation from their colleagues. Indeed the Code of Conduct requires that we work cooperatively and in collaboration with other health care professionals. In practice, however, this can prove problematic.

Doult (1993), writing about the work of the Health Ombudsman in England, suggests that there is little evidence of large-scale refusal to care. It is known (HMSO,

1992) that in 1992 the Health Ombudsman received a total of 1176 formal complaints from users of the health service. Of this number, approximately 17 per cent (198) involved nurses and were concerned with failure to care. Whether such failure was conscious and therefore constituted refusal to care is, however, not known.

Conclusion

This chapter is an attempt to look at caring from different points of view. Not everyone subscribes to the caring ideology of nursing, and such individuals must not be perceived as uncaring. Grounded in our past, our present and presumably our future, there will always be differences in professional opinion as to the nature of nursing, and different ideologies should be able to coexist in nursing. Regardless of the ideology, the process of nursing must be carried out without a single person ever being refused nursing care.

References

Beardshaw V (1981) *Conscientious Objectors at Work. Mental Hospital Nurses — A Case Study.* London: Social Audit.

Brown J, Kitson A and McKnight T (1992) *Challenges in Caring. Explorations in Nursing and Ethics.* London: Chapman and Hall.

Burnard P and Chapman C (1988) *Professional and Ethical Issues in Nursing.* Chichester: John Wiley and Sons.

Doult B (1993) Glare of publicity. *Nursing Standard*, 7 (15): pp. 18–19.

Ellis P (1993) Role of ethics in modern health care, 1. *British Journal of Nursing*, 2 (2): pp. 144–6.

Grundstein A R (1992) Differences in ethical decision making processes among nurses and doctors. *Journal of Advanced Nursing*, 17 (2): pp. 129–37.

HMSO (1992) *Health Service Commissioner for England for Scotland and for Wales Annual Report for 1991–92*. London: HMSO.

Huerta S R and Oddi L F (1992) Refusal to care for patients with human immunodeficiency virus/acquired immunodeficiency syndrome: issues and responses. *Journal of Professional Nursing*, 8 (4): pp. 221–30.

International Council of Nurses (1973) Code for Nurses: Ethical Concepts Applied to Nursing. Geneva: ICN.

Marr J (1992) Morals and ethics in nursing. In N Kenworthy, G Snowley and C Gilling (eds) *Common Foundation Studies in Nursing*. Edinburgh: Churchill Livingstone.

Martin J (1993) Lying to patients: can it ever be justified? *Nursing Standard*, 7 (18): pp. 29–31.

Melia K (1987) *Learning and Working: The Occupational Socialisation of Nurses*. London: Tavistock Publications.

Napier B (1985) Assurances over AIDS are misleading and health staff should be cautious (letter). *Nursing Mirror*, 161: p. 11.

Royal College of Nursing (1976) *Code of Professional Conduct — A Discussion Document*. London: RCN.

Rumbold G (1986) *Ethics in Nursing Practice*. London: Baillière Tindall.

Sampson C (1982) *The neglected ethic. Religious and Cultural Factors in the Care of Patients*. London: McGraw Hill.

Sim J (1992) AIDS, nursing and occupational risk: an ethical analysis. *Journal of Advanced Nursing*, 17 (5): pp. 569–75.

Stockwell F (1984) *The Unpopular Patient*. London: Croom Helm.

Tak Leung Chan T (1993) Black and ethnic minority clients: meeting needs. *Nursing Standard*, 7 (2): pp. 9–14.

Thompson I, Melia K and Boyd K (1988) *Nursing Ethics*. Edinburgh: Churchill Livingstone.

Tschudin V (1986) *Ethics in Nursing: The Caring Relationship*. London: Heinemann.

Tschudin V (1992) *Ethics in Nursing: The Caring Relationship* (2nd edn.). Oxford: Butterworth-Heinemann.

UKCC (1992) *Code of Professional Conduct* (3rd edn.). London: UKCC.

Walsh P (1982) Why I am opposing the doctors. *Nursing Times*, Sept. 22: pp. 1579–80.

Further Reading

Brykczyńska G M (ed.) (1989) *Ethics in Paediatric Nursing*. London: Chapman and Hall.

This book and its contributors provide an excellent resource for exploring ethical dilemmas in caring for children. Neonatal nursing, community care and the child with profound disability are explored, among other topics.

Davis A J and Aroskar M A (1983) *Ethical Dilemmas and Nursing Practice* (2nd edn.). Norwalk, Connecticut: Appleton-Century-Crofts.

This is a very readable book containing a specific chapter on learning disability which should be of interest to nurses in this specialty.

Rowson R H (1990) *An Introduction to Ethics for Nurses*. London: Scutari Press.

This is an excellent introduction to ethics for nurses. The book is divided into two parts. The first part provides an underlying, easy-to-assimilate approach to ethics. The second part applies a number of moral views to a particular decision concerning the management of a patient. Students seeking concrete examples of application will find this very useful.

Steele S M and Harmon V M (1983) *Values Clarification in Nursing* (2nd edn.). Norwalk, Conn.: Appleton-Century-Crofts.

This book explores decision-making in nursing. It is highly relevant to problem-solving in professional situations, especially in the area of ethical dilemmas. It is an interesting and dynamic book which attempts to make bridges between theory and practice.

CHAPTER 2

Withdrawal of Labour

Ann Leedham

Should nurses take industrial action? Is this a political or an ethical decision? Should nurses strike for better pay? Would this not be self-defeating? Are the examples of other countries transferable to the UK?

The author's wide experience of industrial relations gives this chapter a wide scope. She examines research, principles and codes to lead readers through this potential minefield, but does not draw any clear-cut conclusions other than appealing to nurses' individual consciences.

In the UK, nurses are well known for their lack of militancy. The common view of nurses is that they are passive people who put the patient first before any personal gain. However, over the last 20 years, nurses have become more vociferous in their demonstrations regarding their conditions of work and pay, as well as decrying cutbacks in the health service.

Even so, for most nurses any form of industrial action is still unacceptable, and because of this reluctance, it could be argued that nurses have relinquished any bargaining power not only to improve their conditions of work but also to protect the patients' rights.

The main reason nurses give for not taking part in industrial action is that it would harm the very people that they are employed to protect. The ICN, in its *Code for Nurses* (1973), states, 'The fundamental responsibility of the nurse is fourfold: to promote health, to prevent illness, to restore health and to alleviate suffering.' If nurses are to keep to this Code of Conduct which gives them pro-

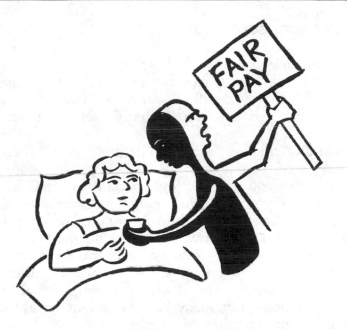

fessional status, any form of industrial action is unacceptable.

   But there is another side to this argument. If others by
their actions prohibit nurses from keeping to a professional
code of conduct, then surely if all avenues have been
explored without effect, nurses may have no choice but
to resort to industrial action. This is the nurses' dilemma:
if they do nothing to improve their lot they are seen as
powerless, but if they take any form of industrial action,
they are likely to be pilloried by both the public and the
government.

   Some nurses who are politically motivated and are
members of radical unions have taken part in aggressive
protests, but the main nurses' unions, for example the
Royal College of Nursing, have consistently refused to
take strike action. In this chapter, we will examine the
arguments surrounding the ethics of industrial action.

Some Facts about Nursing

Firstly, nursing is an essential service; there are approximately 500 000 nurses working in Britain at the present time, and if they were all to withdraw their labour, even for an hour, the cost to the health service would be enormous.

Secondly, nursing may be defined as a vocation, although most people who become nurses see it as a job and not a way of life. The logic behind this definition is that it is mainly women who train to become nurses, and women are often seen to be in the role of self-sacrificing carers. However, for many women there may have been little choice to take up other careers, maybe because at school they were not offered any other opportunities than nursing or teaching. This is not to downgrade either of these professions, but many women might have chosen another avenue had they been offered it.

Finally, as a group, nurses are not very assertive; however, it is a mistake to think that they will passively accept all decisions made by governments concerning themselves and the health service. Over the last 20 years, many nurses have stepped down from their pedestal and entered the political arena, using industrial action to fight for what they believe is right.

What is Meant by Industrial Action?

Industrial action can mean several things, from the complete withdrawal of labour by the workforce to working to rule or agreeing to carry out essential services only. The decision to take industrial action is not taken lightly by most groups of workers, and there is usually more than one factor contributing to the reasons for some form of action being taken. Generally, before decisions are made by the workforce on the type of industrial action to be taken, several months of negotiation with management have taken place. It is the result of the deadlock of negotiations which finally leads workers to the decision to take strike action.

Strike action is not the only method which employees have of expressing their discontent with management, although striking is the most visible and has the greatest impact. However, industrial action does take other forms. At the one end of the continuum, employees can take a grievance out against management which could lead to an industrial tribunal. Other actions may take the form of boycotts, restriction of output, sabotage, absenteeism, high turnover of personnel or mass resignation. Several of these forms of industrial action, such as sabotage, restriction of output, absenteeism and high personnel turnover, may take place on an individual as well as an organised basis and constitute an alternative to collective action. This means that striking itself is not always clear cut. It may involve all the workers or only key people and take the form of refusal to work overtime or to perform a certain process. It may even mean such rigid adherence to the rules that output is stifled.

Nurses have never favoured direct industrial action which places patients at risk, but they have, on certain occasions, been willing to use other forms of indirect industrial action (for example demonstrations and protests outside hospital gates) to bring about changes in their circumstances. However, most nurses have not wished to take part in either direct or indirect action, although that is not to say that they are happy about their pay and conditions of service. It is estimated that approximately 30 000 nurses leave the profession every year. Nurses are in the main female and usually leave for family reasons, but this does not alone account for the fact that few wish to return to the rigours of nursing after a break in service.

There may be many reasons for this; however, a lot of nurses do not feel valued, their pay does not reflect the work they do and they do not, therefore, wish to return to a profession that undervalues them.

Is Industrial Action Effective?

Most nurses believe that even if they resorted to taking widespread industrial action, it would not be that effective. Not only would they lose public sympathy but their action would also lower their professional status. The Royal College of Nursing (RCN) and Royal College of Midwives (RCM) have a 'no strike' rule. They believe that this is a powerful weapon in their negotiations with government about conditions of work and pay for nurses. After all, it would appear very difficult to refuse a group of people who will not take strike action. However, it can also be argued that instead of strengthening nurses, the very fact that they refuse to take action means that governments feel they can ignore this particular group of workers' demands for better pay and conditions of service.

In the 1980s, the Conservative government did much to reduce the power of the unions and was also very vociferous in its claims that strike action never works. The government has always claimed that, in the long run, the workers are the losers. By following this argument to its conclusion, it would be fair to assume that the government would be more likely to reward groups of workers who did not favour industrial action. This has not been the case with the nurses; even though they gained a 15 per cent pay rise in 1988, they have seen their conditions of service deteriorate over the last few years.

Industrial action abroad

In other countries, nurses have not been so reluctant as their British counterparts to take either indirect or direct industrial action. Several times at the end of the 1980s, Canadian nurses took direct industrial action. As a consequence of these strikes, nurses doubled their salary and achieved significant improvements in fringe benefits and working conditions. The union gained a reputation as an effective and powerful collective bargaining agent. Interestingly, the Canadian government subsequently passed legislation to remove the right to strike of all hospital workers. In characteristic defiance, the Canadian nurses' union called a full strike, which led to an unprecedented disruption of the health service. These events led to changes in attitudes of the public policy-makers, and the government announced a 30 million dollar programme of job enhancement for nurses to alleviate some of the work and manpower problems at the root of the union's militancy.

Similarly, in Australia, nurses have struck; they lost much public support but gained in terms of salaries and conditions of service. In the United States, too, nurses have shown themselves to be militant when pushed into a corner.

These groups of nurses mentioned above decided that they could no longer be put in an untenable position. Although they shattered the public perception of nursing, it meant that they were a force which the government of the day could no longer ignore. Public opinion seemed to matter little to these nurses; it seems that they were more concerned about empowerment of nurses and the establishment of nursing rights.

The reason that nurses in other countries are more militant than British nurses can only be surmised. It may be that in these countries women are culturally recognised as a powerful, assertive group or that education is available to a wider group of women, but whatever the reasons for the nurses deciding to take industrial action, the effects have been to strengthen the profession and gain recognition for the work that it does.

The effect of the media

Industrial action may not be the only method nurses have to influence the government. The strongest weapon that British nurses have is the media. Nurses have learnt over the last 20 years to manipulate this particular avenue to highlight the difficulties they face. Most of the big nursing campaigns in the 1970s and 1980s took the form of a high-profiled protest which was given national coverage by the press and on television. The impact of nurses taking to the streets to fight for both the patients' and their own rights ensured that they maintained public support; all the unions, whether they were professional or trade union affiliates, believed that if workers in the health service were ever going to make the government accede to their demands, they had to have the general public on their side.

In conclusion, to be effective and have the greatest impact, industrial action needs to be well organised, but the cost in terms of the harm it may cause the patients and the effect it has on the nurses' standing in society may mean that the end cannot justify the means.

The Unions' Views on Industrial Action

Since 1970, legislation has been passed to control and restrict strikes to specific areas and to control extreme types of industrial action. However, laws are impotent to a certain extent when the relationship between employees and management has broken down to such a degree that there is no alternative but to take direct industrial action.

Whether such action actually works to change government or management minds regarding the demands of the workforce is debatable.

Certainly, the strikes by the miners and ambulance drivers in the 1980s did little to improve their circumstances, and in the end the workers were the losers.

The debate on how effective direct industrial action is in changing the minds of government has caused much dissension among the health unions. The RCN, on the one hand, argues that industrial action has a negative effect on both management and government. As has already been indicated, the RCN has a 'no strike' policy, which it believes is a powerful weapon to use when making demands on government. However, NUPE and COHSE (now jointly with NALGO, Unison) think that industrial action of some sort will not only raise public awareness of the predicament of nurses and the conditions within the health service, but will also effect change by government and management.

The trade union affiliates have encouraged nurses to strike over the years, but the TUC has its own Code of Conduct which does not allow unions to lift emergency cover for essential services without which people may die. Therefore, no union which represents health workers can call an all-out strike. The call for strike action is used more as a threat and as part of a campaign to change working conditions. Protests and lobbying are the only ways in which the unions can make their point. This is why public opinion is so important.

The power of nursing

So, if direct action is not possible, the unions have to rely on the most powerful group, that is nurses, when fighting for the NHS workforce. However, Clay (1987) argues that there are two myths about industrial relations and nurses which need to be disputed. The first is that 'nurses are not powerful as a group in society', and the second is that 'the public always love nurses'.

If nurses did call an all-out strike, it is debatable whether the general public would continue to hold them in such high esteem. However, British public opinion appears to carry some weight, and for this reason, governments have wasted little time during periods of unrest in the health service to inform the public that it is the health workers, especially the nurses, who are behaving irresponsibly in protesting about working conditions.

Even so, as nurses in Britain have not resorted to the use of mass strike action, politicians seem, on the whole, to be complacent about the awesome power and the serious consequences for the health service if nurses were to withdraw their labour or even work to rule. Nurses are key workers in ensuring that patients are cared for 24 hours a day, as well as being the largest group of workers in the NHS, so they are a powerful group in the workplace. However, because nurses do not always assert themselves as a unified group, they do not use this power to good effect. They tend to undervalue themselves, and their low esteem has affected other professional groups and the government's attitude towards them.

Another reason for their apparent lack of power is that nurses have been slow in stepping into the political arena and have not gained a powerful foothold in the political lobbies, as have doctors.

A further problem which has undermined the power of nurses is that nurses form a very disparate group. In 1989, there were nearly 500 000 nurses working in Britain; 64 per cent were qualified professionals, 13 per cent were in training and the remaining 23 per cent were auxiliaries and assistants. However, of the 64 per cent professional group, at least 25 per cent were enrolled nurses. These figures highlight the problem that a person does not have to obtain a registered qualification to be called 'nurse'. This disparity has not gone unnoticed by the government, and this has meant that it has been easier to 'divide and rule' nurses.

Over the last 20 years, one can count on the fingers of one hand the times when nurses have come together to fight for their rights. It has been a slow evolution for nurses to realise their potential in the political arena and to use this power to increase their status in the health service.

Industrial Action — Why is it an Option?

What then are the circumstances which will unite nurses to take some form of industrial action? It appears that ward closures, lack of resources for patients and poor conditions of service, coupled with the failure of the government to increase nurses' pay to a satisfactory level, are the ingredients necessary to bring nurses out on the streets in protest. A quote from *Nursing Times* in 1988 (*Nursing Times*, 1988a) highlights this:

> To-day nurses at the North Middlesex Hospital are taking strike action. Last week NUPE, NALGO and COHSE decided that this was the only way in which they could show the public and the government how they felt about the state of the NHS. Feelings ran strong, but the atmosphere in the wards of the North Middlesex last week was of sadness — not anger.

Rarely has pay been the only reason why nurses have decided to rise up and protest. In all the major campaigns since 1970, it has been a culmination of problems in the health service, affecting both patients and staff, which has driven nurses to take extreme action. It appears that only when nurses feel totally powerless to control changes occurring in the workplace will they decide on radical action. Even then, emergency cover is still maintained.

To take the decision to go on strike is never easy for a group of workers, but if they are not directly harming anyone by their actions, do they have any more right than nurses to take industrial action? Does a nurse's work, by its very nature, preclude any form of industrial action? Here we find the nub of this conundrum: ethically, can any nurse ever withdraw his or her labour?

Have Nurses, as Citizens, the Right to Strike?

Nurses are members of society and therefore, it can be argued, have the same rights as all citizens in a democratic society. Do their qualifications, then, negate their rights as citizens to take part in any form of industrial action which may harm the very people they are supposed to protect?

As citizens, the constraints and pressures of everyday working life are common to all those in employment. One of the questions that faces working people concerns the moral problems associated with the need to take industrial action, either in defence of one's job or in an attempt to maintain comparative living standards and working conditions.

Nurses or any medical workers who decide to go on strike know that this may result in someone either suffering or dying. Brecher (1986) argues that adopting the position that no medical worker should strike must apply to *everyone*, especially to those whose power over life and death is the greatest, or it does not apply at all. If someone dies as a result of a nurse striking, does that mean that that individual nurse behaved immorally? Brecher argues, on the one hand, that human life is either so special or so important that there are no circumstances at all in which it is possible to justify not doing everything possible to preserve it. Alternatively, writes Brecher, a particular group, because of the essential nature of its work, is morally correct in taking strike action because the end justifies the means.

Brecher goes on to say that we all hold the first view, because if nothing can justify any omission, let alone commission, which leads to the death of a human being, prime ministers, MPs, civil servants and all citizens are responsible for maintaining life. Nurses are part of that shared responsibility and therefore have the same rights as any other citizen, while governments and ordinary citizens are just as directly responsible as nurses for ensuring that people are cared for. For example, as a result of government policy, at least one fewer kidney machine is in service than it would be possible to have provided; one person died of cancer last week who need not have died had resources been differently allocated; one more person in Africa has died of starvation than would have died if an individual had sent £5 to a charity. If nothing can justify any omission, just one avoidable death is morally culpable. This view is obviously not espoused by many people, especially politicians.

The second view, that the end justifies the means, is more difficult to uphold. For example, if a group of nurses decide that the only choice that they have is to take some form of industrial action, which means leaving a ward of patients, can they really justify this action if one person dies, even though management may give in to their demands, and conditions of work are improved to such an extent that patients are much better cared for in the long run? Do the means justify the end? There is general agreement that the number of people who are killed annually by road traffic is worth the benefits resulting from the mobility made possible by cars. However, few would deny that the number of deaths ought to be reduced — although not at any cost. After all, it would be possible to reduce road casualty numbers to zero by banning road traffic. Presumably we, or most of us, would agree that the result-ant harm would outweigh the moral benefit.

Proximity and contractual obligation

Brecher (1986) goes on to argue that this alleged responsi-bility comes in two closely connected guises: proximity and contractual obligation. He gives the example of what he means by proximity as follows: if you or I see an accident, we have a moral obligation to do what we can to help, simply from being there. By the same token, the nurse has an obligation to help because she or he is there. All the talk of ministerial responsibility or citizen's respon-sibility is, at best, entirely artificial because ministers are in Whitehall and citizens are at home; it is the *nurse* who is there. To go on strike is to avoid that proximity; surely, those who have voluntarily put themselves in a position of proximate responsibility have a moral obligation not to avoid it. After all, no-one is forced to become a nurse. Those who do are therefore under a contractual obligation to perform the duties they have agreed to undertake.

If such workers are under a special contractual obligation because of the nature of the work they have voluntarily undertaken to perform, the question is whether they are also under some obligation to continue being such workers for life. If, for example, nurses are under special obligation not to strike, are they also, by the same argument, under special obligation not to give up their job? Brecher argues that this would be nonsense, for if they were, one might reasonably ask on what grounds anyone should be expected to become a nurse. Why should any particular person be expected to place her- or himself under such an onerously special obligation?

Brecher does not see how the question of ceasing to be a nurse differs from that of a nurse going on strike in respect of specific consequences of such action, namely a person's death. Whether or not the likelihood of certain specific consequences being set against others constitutes good moral grounds for not ceasing to be a nurse is one and the same question as whether it constitutes good moral grounds for not going on strike.

One can extend this argument further and ask whether society and government regard the jobs of specific health workers, such as nurses, as so special that they are morally obliged to ensure that special responsibilities that nurses undertake receive special benefits. Just the opposite happens in the National Health Service. Many nurses are undervalued, underpaid and working in very poor conditions. Therefore it could be said that the government have reneged on their contract, so nurses have the right to take industrial action to make the government recognise their responsibility. However, can the government be held responsible if we accept that a nurse has the same rights as any citizen, especially the right to choose? By the time they qualify and register with the UKCC, nurses are aware of what their work entails, so they cannot argue that they have been forced into nursing without any prior knowledge. Because nurses choose to nurse, do they then abdicate all rights to industrial action because of their understanding of the nature of their work? In other words, because a nurse chooses to care for people who are in need through no fault of their own, does this factor preclude the nursing profession from taking any form of industrial action? This concept is strongly linked with notions of professionalism.

Professionalism

Wan, Sullivan and Christensen (1991) found a strong feeling of professionalism existing among nurses regarding their sense of duty, obligation and standards of care for

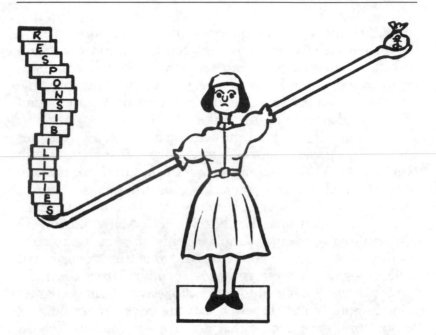

those using hospital services. He discovered that whichever
union the nurses belong to, there exists a strong professional ethic which is juxtaposed with the spectrum of
attitudes towards industrial action, ranging from total
rejection of action at one extreme to strike action at the
other. These variables appear as a result of the diversity of
nurses in the NHS.

Wan, Sullivan and Christens (1991) found that among
lower grades, males (only 10 per cent of nurses in Britain),
younger staff and those working in psychiatric hospitals,
there was a greater willingness to take direct industrial
action. We can only surmise the reasons which lay behind
this and conclude that those nurses working in the lower
grades are the worst paid and work in very difficult conditions. They also do not have the autonomy of nurses who
work in higher grades. This leads to dissatisfaction with
their role, and this may be one of the reasons why they
are more willing to take strike action. Additionally, the

expectations of male nurses tend to be higher than those of female nurses: they expect to work for most of their lives and they see nursing much more as a career, whereas many women view nursing as a part-time job which they can move in and out of depending on their family circumstances. Obviously, this is not to say that women have fewer concepts of professional status than men.

Since the days of Florence Nightingale, nurses have fought to develop nursing as a profession. Over the decades, they have developed a body of knowledge and standards of practice which are unique to nursing. A great leap forward was made in 1979 when Parliament passed the Nurses, Midwives and Health Visitors Act. The recognition of nursing as a profession has not been won easily, and for this reason nurses are very reluctant to bring the profession into disrepute. Maybe the very thing they strove to gain will prevent nurses from securing a more powerful base in the political arena.

Do Nurses Have the Right to Choose?

Freedom of choice is central to the dilemma of whether strike action for nurses is right or wrong. Choice is also linked to another aspect of freedom — freedom to help the patient to choose. Thus the nurse–patient relationship is based on advocacy, assuming that nurses believe that they have the right to choose and that that right is accepted by society. In theory, the empowerment of the patient is increased as a result of the nurses' actions, but is this true in reality? Nurses working in the health care field can see the quality of patient care suffer as a result of incompetent health professionals, inflexible institutional policies and an overburdened health delivery system that cannot meet the demands made upon it. Therefore, nurses' choice regarding the delivery of care they give to the patient is reduced.

Nurses who recognise a dehumanisation and debasement of patient care are disturbed by their acquiescence and participation in the process but often feel incapable of effecting changes or improving situations. The main reason for this is that nurses are not in the position to change policies which affect patient care. If this is the case, can nurses be given the responsibility of being the patients' advocate? This can lead to what has been termed as professional disillusionment, reality shock and moral distress (Jameton, 1984).

These three problems relate to the sense of frustration, sadness and anger that nurses feel about their practice. Of the three, moral distress emphasises the ethical component of the situation, which occurs when nurses know the right thing to do 'but institutional constraints make it nearly impossible to pursue the right course of action' (Jameton, 1984). Therefore, the frustration that nurses feel because they do not have the power or autonomy to make decisions regarding their work may make them feel less morally responsible for the outcome of their action. Nurses thus feel that they have no power or control over their actions. In frustration, they may consider industrial action. In considering nurses as advocates for patients, advocacy can be linked to the ethical principle of individual freedom, and within that freedom there has to be choice, but if nurses do not feel they have choice, arguably they cannot be the patients' advocate.

Empowerment and autonomy

There are two issues here: empowerment and autonomy. However, if the system is so inflexible that the individuals within the health service who are actually delivering patient care do not feel empowered or autonomous, this can eventually lead to 'professional disobedience', which was defined by Abrams (1980) as 'a refusal of nurses to carry out immoral or unsafe orders from authorities higher in the health care hierarchy.'

Many nurses have been reluctant to recognise the independent nature of their practice. As Ritter, Crulcich and McEntegart (1982) put it:

> A lack of knowledge and assertiveness, a fear of failure, a fear of assuming responsibility and a fear to be held accountable for their actions, fosters the development and maintenance of passive dependence.

The unwillingness of many nurses to assume responsibility for decision-making and the lack of support for nurses who try to increase their level of autonomy has limited nursing's efforts to achieve parity in the health care system. There are many reasons for this, the first of them being that 90 per cent of nurses are women who have learned to be passive and obedient to the male medical hierarchy. This has meant that nurses have been reluctant to take responsibility for decisions. The strength of the medical hierarchy has had a fundamental effect on the nursing profession. 'Because the doctor ordered it' has meant, then, that nurses have been reluctant to assume the responsibility of nursing care, which is definitely different from the work carried out by the doctor.

Nurses have to decide what is meant by nursing care and make sure that they alone are responsible for the delivery of that care. There are many areas of nursing practice overlapping with medical diagnosis and treatment which will obviously be affected by the physician's authority; no area of nursing practice is truly independent. However, legal precedent has established the necessity of nurses challenging the treatment of patients by physicians when the basic standards are not met (Walker, 1983).

Another area which has undermined the nurses' autonomy is that nurses feel primarily responsible to the hospital rather than to the patient. It is often said that nurses are just following hospital policy, and a great emphasis is placed by managers at high level on policies being followed to the letter, disciplinary procedures often being used if policies are broken. Such an inflexible approach to this task-orientated idea of patient care needs to be challenged if nurses are going to be patients' advocates.

As the perception of the nurses' responsibility to the patient has developed since the late 1960s, the power of the physician has shrunk and that of the patient has grown. Patients have now new-found rights, for example privacy, confidentiality, autonomy and respect. The advocacy role focuses almost entirely on the patient's right to autonomy, assuming that autonomy is the most important point in patient welfare (Brody, 1988). However, nurses often confuse the advocacy role with defending or rescuing the client, which can foster patient dependency and low self-esteem.

Nurses often believe that they are the only health professionals working in the patients' best interests. Brody argues that:

> the role of the patient advocate is to inform the patient and then sit back and let the patient decide for himself or herself without coercion, threat or persuasion. The values and wishes of the patient become the deciding factors in determining nursing actions.

Kohnke (1982) in his book *Advocacy: Risk and Reality*, states that 'Judgment is not part of the role of the advocate; the advocate's duty is only to ensure the right of free will or free choice.' But is the nurse the only person who can be the advocate?

If patients have the freedom to choose from the information they are given, does it always have to be the nurse who gives them that information? To follow this argument to its logical conclusion one would say that nurses are not essential in the role of advocate; therefore, if they were to

take industrial action, patients would not necessarily die
or be harmed. Brody (1988) argues that some nurses would
prefer to avoid actively participating in decision-making,
in the mistaken belief that this lack of participation
removes them from any moral responsibility for their
actions. They fail to see that they have already made a
choice — a choice not to choose — and that they therefore
cannot escape moral responsibility for their own practice.
If we accept that nurses do not always accept responsibility
for the care they deliver, ethically they cannot be held
responsible if they take strike action.

Professional collectiveness

Let us return to this concept of professional disobedience.
Disobedience is usually a collective activity:

> Throughout history, when men (sic) have disobeyed or
> rebelled, they have done so, by and large, as members
> or representatives of a group. They have claimed not merely
> that they are free to disobey but they are obligated to do
> so. (Walzer, 1967)

'Professional disobedience' can therefore only occur when
people feel empowered enough to stand up for their rights.

When people choose to become nurses, they enter a
profession which has established standards of ethical conduct. The professional collective provides the forum for
debate and resolution of practice issues and the setting of
standards for practice and evaluation. When nurses do not
meet this established professional level of conduct, they
have breached their duty as nurses. Equally, however, when
they are unable to reach that level of professionalism
because of the inflexible hierarchy, it can be argued that
the hierarchy is in breach of its duty to the nurses; thus it
can be proposed that nurses should be able to take some
form of industrial action to achieve their aims.

Abrams (1980) states that during a professional dispute, a nurse chooses not to conform to the orders of superiors because the professional standards developed by the nursing community for her or his public role as a nurse are being compromised. Professional disobedience is tied to the duties a nurse has in her or his public role, and shared standards of practice are justified for its use. As a result of financial constraints, hospitals are forced to close wards and reduce the number of nurses working with the patients, so nurses are justified in taking some form of industrial action to highlight the plight of the patients.

Only through collective action can the profession seek and maintain control of its practice in order to guarantee the quality of its service to the public. Nurses need to develop an understanding of collective support of the individual; for example, if one group of nurses decides, for ethical reasons, that direct industrial action is inevitable, they need the collective support of the profession to withdraw their labour in order to reach their goal. This can be seen as 'professional action' which leads to improvement in standards of practice.

Other Ethical Approaches to Industrial Action

Seedhouse (1988) would affirm that the controversy of whether nurses can withdraw their labour or not can be argued in two ways — basing decisions about how to act, firstly, on the assessment of the likely consequences or outcomes of actions, and, secondly, on beliefs about certain duties taken to be fundamental to the very idea of morality. For example, the utilitarian approach assesses the worth or morality of what people do either by looking at the actual results, and so judging morality in retrospect, or by calculating the likely future outcomes of their actions. Therefore, if taking any form of industrial action leads to the happiness of a great number of people, it could be said that, morally, industrial action is correct and the proper approach to effecting change.

But here we find the dichotomy: who decides whether industrial action is good or bad? It certainly depends on from which perspective one is arguing the moral nature of industrial action. For the government, and in turn management, industrial action is wrong. Nothing can be gained from withdrawing labour, but workers can justify as right and proper the decision to take industrial action because it is their right to decide whether they work or not. If one takes the utilitarian approach, the only ethical action which is acceptable is that which produces the greatest happiness or pleasure for humankind as a whole.

Seedhouse (1988) also discusses the ethical theory known as deontology. This theory states that what matters most is not the result, but the fact that the person acted according to a perceived duty and intended that some good should come about. The philosopher who advocates deontology might argue that certain principles, i.e. truth-telling and promise-keeping, are fundamental to morality, and that to be a moral person, there is a moral duty always to abide by these principles, whatever the consequences. For example, if a nurse is faced with having to tell a patient the truth about his or her medical condition, even though this may produce more misery than happiness, it is the nurse's moral duty to act in such a way.

The central feature of deontology is the concept of integrity. All decisions should generally be made by referring to honest principles rather than being based on expedient calculation. For the deontologist, a nurse could, in certain circumstances, withdraw his or her labour if it meant standing for principles which were being undermined by other parties. However, Abrams (1980) would argue that professional non-compliance should never occur when it could break a major ethical principle. For example, if being disobedient could cause harm to a patient, it is not justifiable.

Brody (1988) argues that ethical principles such as autonomy and beneficence often conflict in practice, and any nursing action, including professional disobedience, may therefore have to break an ethical principle. At this point, principles supporting different courses of action must be judged and prioritised. However, professional disobedience should never occur when it would break the principle of non-maleficence, the most basic and inviolable principle. Because the justification for professional disobedience lies in the nurse's prime responsibility to the patient, a nurse cannot justify disobedience when the patient could be harmed.

Does this mean that nurses never have the freedom to decide what is best for themselves and, in turn, their patients? Within all these arguments, we are seeing that nurses are expected to behave in a way that puts them above other workers. However, if their situation in the workplace is intolerable, can they really be expected to reach the high standards which society, the profession and the establishment demand of them?

Do Nurses have the Right to Strike?

So far we have established that nurses do have rights, as do any citizens living in a democracy, but their rights concerning strike action are still debatable.

All nurses have to register with the UKCC which lays down a Code of Professional Conduct (UKCC, 1992) as a guideline to nursing practice. The dilemma that faces nurses, implicit within the UKCC Code of Professional Conduct, is that if nurses take strike action, they are no longer acting in a manner which safeguards and promotes the interests of the patients. Thus, they can technically be struck off the Register if they do not adhere to the professional Code of Conduct.

In 1988 the UKCC was put to the test regarding a small minority of nurses who took strike action. In February 1988, nurses' anger about their conditions in the health service erupted into a widescale protestation, and strike action was called by the TUC unions. There was pressure on the RCN to revoke its Rule 12, and a ballot was held in April 1988, resulting in an overwhelming vote to retain Rule 12 (the no-strike rule). However, many nurses were still dissatisfied with the RCN as they believed that the ballot had been biased. Throughout 1988, there were several organised protests, but strike action was only seen to be taken in controlled circumstances. Nurses belonging to the RCN covered the clinical areas for those nurses in NUPE and COHSE who wished to take direct action.

Controversy broke out in January 1988 over the UKCC's decision on industrial action. They issued a statement regarding any industrial action which was as follows (*Nursing Times*, 1988b):

1 The UKCC Code of Professional Conduct 1984 for the nurse, midwife and health visitor applies to each and every person on the UKCC professional register.
2 The Code of Professional Conduct is the major part of the background against which the allegations of misconduct are judged.
3 The introductory paragraph of the Code emphasises that the interests of the patients should dominate over those of the profession.
4 Clauses 1 and 2 of the Code deliberately emphasise each nurse's personal accountability:
> Clause 1: Act always in such a way as to promote and safeguard the well being and interests of patients/clients.
> Clause 2: Ensure that no action or omission on his/her part or within his/her sphere of

influence is detrimental to the condition or
safety of patients/clients.

5   Any citizen has the right to allege misconduct against
    any nurse and all such allegations must be investigated
    and judged through the group process of the profession's
    legislation to determine whether the person who is the
    subject of allegations should lose or retain the right to
    practise. The fact that the individual is participating in a
    group or an industrial action does not dilute or eliminate
    personal accountability.

6   The quoted clauses from the Code indicate that the
    UKCC is concerned that no actions or omissions be
    detrimental to the conditions or safety of patients,
    irrespective of the reason.

7   Any person whose name is on the Council's register
    should recognise, as a matter of self interest, that they
    are personally accountable for their actions or omissions
    and should seriously consider their position and measure
    any such proposed actions or omissions against the text
    of the Code of Professional Conduct.

This statement from the UKCC intimated that any nurse
who took any form of industrial action would put his or
her registration into jeopardy.

There are two other points which are worth noting.
Firstly, the UKCC asserts that nurses are personally
accountable for their conduct, and therefore it is a personal
decision if they wish to take industrial action. Secondly,
the UKCC would only investigate such action if the nurse
in question was reported to it, whereupon it would consider the circumstances in which the industrial action was
taken.

The UKCC, as the representative body of nursing, does
not favour any form of indirect or direct industrial action,
whatever the circumstances. The UKCC talks about the
individual's responsibility but fails to address issues of collective responsibility. After all, industrial action, by its very
nature, has to be a collective act, so can an individual be

held responsible for the actions of a group? We have established that industrial action is only taken as a last resort; therefore, if conditions of work are so intolerable that nurses cannot achieve the demands which are laid down in the professional Code of Conduct, are they not justified in taking industrial action which will improve their conditions of employment? If the UKCC refuses to support nurses in this, is not then the UKCC to be held responsible for not acting as the nurses' advocate?

The unions and the UKCC

Most of the support for nurses in their quest to improve their situation has come from the professional unions like the RCN and RCM. That is not to say that these unions have agreed with strike action. They have argued that indirect and direct industrial action would be detrimental to the profession. However, the difference between the RCN and RCM and the UKCC is that the RCN and RCM are professional trade unions which nurses can choose to be members of. The Colleges represent qualified nurses, midwives and health visitors as well as student nurses, both on an individual and collective basis. The role of the unions is to champion the cause of nurses as well as developing nurses professionally and educationally. It is for the unions to find the middle road where they can put pressure to bear on the establishment to change the conditions of service under which nurses work.

   In conclusion, is there a difference between the UKCC and unions like the RCN and the RCM, and do they have different responsibilities to nurses and the nursing profession? In the first instance, the UKCC was set up by an Act of Parliament. All qualified nurses in Britain are members of the UKCC, bound by a Code of Professional Conduct which is laid down by the profession. The RCN and RCM are professional trade unions which nurses can

choose to belong to. It is for the members to decide whether
they wish to strike or not, and it is the members who
choose whether the union has a 'no strike' clause within
its rules. To remove the rule, members have to be balloted.
Clay (1987) argues that a true professional is a person who
always puts duty first, and it is for a trade union to seek
to ensure that its members are never put into the position
of having to choose between the patient or strike action.

Over the last few years, there has been increasing pressure from certain quarters to rescind the 'no strike' policy.
One could argue that there is no longer any point in
having a 'no strike' policy as the UKCC Code of Professional Conduct controls whether or not nurses take
industrial action. However, the RCN has always argued
that the 'no strike' rule is about choice. Nurses choose
not to strike because they are professionals who put the
patient first. This argument can be used as a powerful
political weapon in the negotiations with government
about pay and conditions of service.

The 'no strike' rule is used, more than anything else, as
a statement. It stands for a professional and caring attitude
which is an integral part of nursing. It also tells the world
that nurses are professionals and will always put their
patients first. It shows the general public that, whatever
happens, nurses will not let them down, and it can be
used as a political tool against the establishment. After all,
it is very difficult to lose patience with a union that does
not have a policy of industrial action. How successful the
'no strike' rule is in influencing government is disputed
by the more militant unions. They argue that it is because
they are willing to take direct action that governments are
prepared to change their minds.

Professionalism and industrial action could be reconciled
by demonstration rather than complete stoppage. Although
there were strikes in 1988, RCN members made sure that
they covered for their NUPE and COHSE colleagues.

Because patients were protected, the nurses' actions attracted a high media profile.

The relationship that the professional trade unions have with the UKCC is peculiar in so far as the nurses who are members of the trade union are also members of the UKCC, so it could be argued that both bodies are one and the same. The UKCC is concerned about standards of nursing practice and individual accountability, whereas the unions are more concerned with the collective response of nurses to the changes in practice which are enforced on them by government decision. The arguments surrounding individual accountability and collective responsibility are extremely complex. However, by their very nature, trade unions are representative of a collective group and this is where their power lies, whereas a professional governing body, in the nurses' case the UKCC, is concerned with the individual's ability to keep to the collective rules governing the profession. Both unions and professional bodies can apply pressure on the establishment to effect change in different ways.

Conclusion

Industrial action is a complex topic. It is not a matter of saying that it is wrong to take strike action because to take that action means harming another human being; industrial action and the right to choose are interlinked. Nurses choose to nurse and, as a result of that choice, could be expected in all conscience never to take any form of industrial action. However, as members of society, nurses have the same democratic rights as any citizen, and therefore are not precluded from taking strike action. Nurses are the patients' advocate, which also means that they could never take any form of action which would harm patients. However, advocacy and freedom are synonymous and it could be argued that nurses, to be proper advocates of patients, have freedom of choice, and therefore, in certain instances, any form of industrial action is ethically right. If, as a result of any form of industrial action, nurses are able to improve conditions of service, which will improve patient care, it could be said that industrial action is acceptable.

Industrial action is very much up to the individual's conscience; however, by its very nature, industrial action has to be a collective act. So can the individual be held responsible for the actions of a group of people? Under the UKCC Code of Professional Conduct, the answer is 'yes'. If one accepts the rights of the citizen, the answer is 'no'.

However, even if nurses can justify that industrial action is acceptable in certain instances, can they really justify to themselves and the UKCC that the actual act of withdrawing their labour is acceptable behaviour for nurses?

References

Abrams N (1980) Moral responsibility in nursing. In S F Spicker and S Gadow (eds) *Nursing: Images and Ideals*. New York: Springer Publishing.

Brecher R (1986) Health workers' strikes: A rejoinder rejected. *Journal of Medical Ethics*, 12(1): pp. 40–2.

Brody J (1988) *Professional disobedience in nursing: the moral duty to disobey*. In E Kelly (ed.) *Professional Ethics in Health Care Services*. London: University Press of America.

Clay T (1987) *Nurses, Power & Politics*. London: Heinemann Nursing.

International Council of Nurses (1973) *Code for Nurses: Ethical Concepts Applied to Nursing*. Geneva: ICN.

Jameton A (1984) *Nursing Practice: The Ethical Isues*. Englewood Cliffs, NJ: Prentice-Hall.

Kohnke M F (1982) *Advocacy: Risk and Reality*. St Louis: Mosby.

Nursing Times (1988a) Nurses at the North Middlesex, 84 (5): pp. 16–17.

Nursing Times (1988b) Industrial Action: UKCC statement, 84 (4): p. 21.

Ritter T, Crulcich M and McEntegart A (1982) Nursing practice: An amalgam of dependence, independence and interdependence. In J C McClosky and H K Grace (eds) *Current Issues in Nursing*. Boston: Blackwell Scientific Publications.

Seedhouse D (1988) *Ethics: The Heart of Health Care*. Chichester: John Wiley and Sons.

UKCC (1992) *Code of Professional Conduct* (3rd edn.). London: UKCC.

Walker D J (1983) Legal rights and responsibilities of the nurse. In N L Chaska (ed.) *The Nursing Profession: A Time to Speak*. New York: McGraw Hill.

Walzer M (1967) The obligation to disobey. *Ethics*, 77: pp. 163–74.

Wan D, Sullivan T and Christensen I (1991) *Nurses in the National Health Service. Health Manpower Management*, 17 (3): pp. 22–7.

CHAPTER 3

Whistleblowing

Maureen Eby

One of the 'side effects' of ethical caring is the personal cost sometimes paid by the carers. Whistleblowers have become more common and also more feared. Who dares to care ethically?

This chapter leads the reader through a clear and concise discussion of the origins of whistleblowing and the costs and consequences of any actions in the light of ethical principles. It ends with a conclusion which every potential whistleblower should read.

Whistleblowing is an ancient art of bringing to light wrongdoings in any area of life. Throughout history, individuals have fought heroic battles against insurmountable odds to reveal and right the wrongs of tyrants, whether mythical or real. Robin Hood, the son of the Earl of Locksley, who was accompanying King Richard the Lionheart in the Crusades — even though a purported legend of 14th century England — sought to reveal the treacherous corruption of Prince John, the Regent, along with Baron Guy of Gisborne, Oswald Montdragon, Counsellor to Prince John, and, of course, the Sheriff of Nottingham, Robin Hood's guardian (Fraser, 1971). Robin's adventures, though they are exciting tales of honesty, courage, fidelity and truth, also document treachery, deceit, betrayal and corruption.

A Case History

Mary reported for night shift to discover again that, with sickness and vacancies, she only had an auxiliary to work with during the night. Just the two of them for a 31-bed acute medical ward, with two patients in isolation. This had now been the usual staffing complement for over three weeks, and despite her raising this issue with the ward sister and night sister, with the half-promise of some relief at supper, no-one ever came to assist. Mary was despairing. How could she and an auxiliary meet all these patients' needs during the night? How could she comfort those who needed it, turn those who needed regular pressure area care (which was most of the 31 patients) and keep them all toileted and dry throughout the night? Where was the time for caring?

By now, Mary was beyond rationalising away this lack of staff. For three weeks, she had coped with this overwhelming situation, feeling quite isolated on nights as she was the only staff nurse on the ward and never had the luxury of leaving the ward to see other staff at supper time. She wondered how the others were coping since vacancies were quite high in her hospital, although they never seemed to advertise for staff. Bank nurses appeared to be a relic of the past, as were agency nurses. Just what was happening? This time, if I ever make it through this night, I must confront Sister about this, she vowed.

Sister was late arriving the next morning, but Mary waited. This just can't be right, Mary thought. Patients are entitled to have their needs met, but how can they be if there aren't enough of us? Surely, the Code of Conduct says something about the primacy of meeting patients' needs. I'll start with that.

However, when Sister did arrive she was quite flustered. Mary was too tired to notice and just launched into her carefully orchestrated speech about the primacy of patients' needs and their not being met due to staffing difficulties. Sister listened and finally asked whether Mary had been documenting this or discussing it with anyone else. 'No' said Mary, 'I haven't had the chance'. 'Well', said Sister, 'I think you should forget it. You've only been a staff nurse now for seven months. No-one is going to listen to someone who hasn't got experience behind them. Surely the problems you are experiencing are a reflection of your inexperience and your inability to prioritise and organise your time. If I were you, I wouldn't let anyone else know you can't cope! It wouldn't look good for promotion.'

'But, Sister, it's not a question of prioritising needs. Surely everyone is entitled to comfort, caring and a dry bed for the night' exclaimed Mary, now getting quite angry at the insinuation that she couldn't cope. 'Look', said Sister, herself now quite angry, 'do you want to be known as a whistleblower? Do you want your new career to be finished before it's even started? Keep on the way you're going and I can guarantee you that it will!' With that, Sister got up and left. Mary, both hurt and angry, just sat in Sister's office with tears rolling down her cheeks. 'What have I done', she thought. 'I didn't come into nursing for this, I came because I wanted to care for people — those who needed the skills and knowledge I've been educated to give. How can I achieve this without support and help? I know it's not a question of my inability to cope, and what's Sister called me — a whistleblower! What's that, and wasn't it a threat about my career being finished before it even started? Can she do that? What can I do next? Whom can I turn to? Maybe Sister's right; I don't hear the other nurses complaining about the staffing. Are they coping? Is it really just me? Am I not coping? But why call me a whistleblower, whatever that is?'

With that Mary got up and left. At least, she thought, I have the next seven days off to think things through.

The Background to Whistleblowing

Does the scenario in the case history above sound familiar? Unfortunately, nurses are experiencing situations like this more and more frequently; to see this one only needs to look at the RCN's Whistleblow Scheme, which was

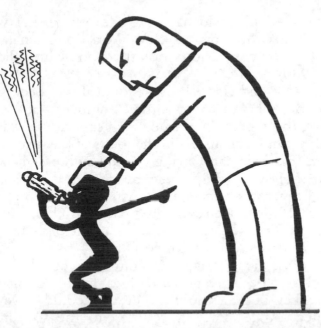

launched in May 1991. From its inception until March 1992, over 100 letters detailing similar incidents had been sent. All these letters dealt with the recurrent theme of 'a lack of resources and a new management culture' (RCN 1992). Perhaps for some this was the first time nurses had actually heard the word 'whistleblower', and even those who had were not exactly certain what it meant.

The ethical concepts existing today are the same as they were for the knights and barons of history, although these may have been replaced with managers and presidents of industry and organisations. Within the last 20 years, there has been an increase in cases of whistleblowing and a resultant increase in the challenges these individuals have faced in overcoming the obstacles placed before them. Some of these people have become legends in their own right and immortalised in cinema and books, for example Karen Silkwood who exposed unsafe working conditions in a plutonium factory and was found dead at the wheel

of her car — an 'accident' — as she was on her way to
testify. Frank Serpico, a New York policeman who
exposed police corruption, was ostracised by his colleagues
(Bok, 1980).

But some individuals' lives could have been saved.
Roger Boisjoly and two other engineers at Morton
Thiokol, Inc. repeatedly warned their superiors and NASA
officials about inadequacies in the joints of the space shuttle
booster, in which the O-rings would stiffen at low tem-
peratures. However, despite these warnings, the space shuttle Challenger was launched in low temperature on January
28th 1986. It exploded soon after take-off, killing all seven
astronauts. This was spectacularly captured on television
for the world to see in stunned horror.

The subsequent Rogers Commission concluded that
the explosion occurred because of seal failure in one of the
solid rocket booster's joints. Yet this could have been
prevented. Roger Boisjoly testified to the Commission
that this knowledge had been made known repeatedly to
officials of both Morton Thiokol and NASA, yet no action
was taken. The outcome of the Commission's report was
that NASA created a position of associate administrator
for safety, reliability and quality assurance, who now had
the authority to stop shuttle launchings in similar circumstances; Roger Boisjoly resigned from his position with
Morton Thiokol, due to hostile pressure (Boisjoly, Curtis
and Mellican, 1989; Florman, 1989; Fitzgerald, 1990).

The word 'whistleblowing' is relatively new to the
modern vocabulary and has been defined by Bok (1984) as
the act of disclosing information, based on an individual's
expertise and insider knowledge of the organisation or
profession, which calls attention to negligence, abuses
or dangers that threaten the public interest. It stems from
the world of sport and refers to the referee blowing the
whistle to stop play when a foul is suspected or observed.
Thus a whistleblower within an organisation, whether it

be industry or the National Health Service, is in effect blowing the whistle to stop play within his or her own team or organisation when a perceived wrongdoing or bureaucratic violation, e.g. inefficiency, incompetency, denial of respect to others, abuse of authority, and/or immoral, ineffective or inefficient policies, has occurred (Fiesta, 1990).

Whistleblowing is a multilayered concept and cannot be viewed in simplistic terms as it has both positive and negative attributes. As such, it becomes a very complex concept to analyse; thus when an individual is caught in a whistleblowing dilemma, much thought needs to be given to all the implications of this concept before any action can be considered. Bok (1980) has identified three elements within whistleblowing that need careful examination: dissent, breach of loyalty and accusation. However, these three elements form only part of the wider concept of whistleblowing, and as such any discussion of whistleblowing must include an examination of the following four ethical concepts:

- Accountability.
- Loyalty or fidelity.
- Justice.
- Truth or veracity.

Accountability

Accountability is an ethical concept that has risen to prominence as nursing has gained in professionalism (see Chapter 5 in *Ethics – Nurses and Patients*). To be accountable means to be able to explain not only one's actions and/ or omissions but also one's choices and their concomitant decision-making process. Accountability has become enshrined within the UKCC's Code of Professional Conduct

(UKCC, 1992) as it is stated as part of the stem to each
of the 16 clauses contained within the Code. As Mary (in
the above case history) assumed, the Code contains several
clauses which she could rightly use in supporting her
concerns over the low staffing levels on nights:

- *Clause 1* — 'act always in such a manner as to promote and safeguard the interests and well-being of
  patients and clients'.
- *Clause 2* — 'ensure that no action or omission on
  your part, or within your sphere of responsibility, is
  detrimental to the interests, condition or safety of
  patients and clients'.
- *Clause 4* — 'acknowledge any limitations in your
  knowledge and competence and decline any duties
  or responsibilities unless able to perform them in a
  safe and skilled manner'.
- *Clause 11* — 'report to an appropriate person or
  authority, having regard to the physical, psychological
  and social effects on patients and clients, any circumstances in the environment of care which could jeop-
  ardise standards of practice'.
- *Clause 12* — 'report to an appropriate person or
  authority any circumstances in which safe and appropriate care for patients and clients cannot be
  provided'.
- *Clause 13* — 'report to an appropriate person or
  authority where it appears that the health or safety
  of colleagues is at risk, as such circumstances may
  compromise standards of practice and care'.

Thus, using the Code, Mary had reported her concerns
to an appropriate person, i.e. the ward sister. As such, Mary
was exercising not only her professional accountability but
also her accountability to her employer, the hospital, to
which the ward sister was also accountable. Of equal
importance was the fact that Mary was being accountable

to herself, and, as Hirschman (1970) describes, Mary elected to confront the problem by speaking out rather than by leaving the organisation or remaining silent, thus not placing self-interest or loyalty to the organisation above her concerns for her patients' welfare. 'Each registered nurse, midwife and health visitor shall act, at all times, in such a manner as to: safeguard and promote the interests of individual patients and clients; serve the interests of society; justify public trust and confidence; and uphold and enhance the good standing and reputation of the profession' (UKCC, 1992). Thus, Mary was being accountable on all three levels: to herself, to her employer and to her profession.

It is interesting to note that in 1991–92, the UKCC reported that the number of proven cases of nurse managers abusing their management position (a total of 34) had increased nearly two and a half times from the previous year (a total of 14), and about seven times from the year before (a total of 5). Abuse of management position now ranks third with physical and other abuses of patients and is still ahead in the league table of misconduct (Mason, 1992).

So whistleblowing can be viewed as a mechanism of accountability. It is certainly seen as 'after-the-fact' accountability, as the individual is usually bringing to public light facts after they have occurred (Jos, 1991). However, it may well be the case that the individual tried, within the internal mechanisms of the organisation, to bring to light these facts prior to an incident occurring, such as the case with Mary, above. Mary was bringing to the sister's attention the effects of low staffing on the night shift and its implications for safe and competent patient care. She was, in Batey and Lewis's (1982) words, being 'proactively accountable' in that she was attempting to initiate some action based on her accountability of the low staffing levels on nights.

The sister, on the other hand, is seen as being 'reactively

accountable' in that it appears that she is going to put
off any action until an incident forces her to recount
retrospectively and defensively to those external to the
service, e.g. the Coroner's Office, should an increase in
patient death rate go unnoticed for a prolonged period of
time due to low staffing levels, or should a patient die as
a result of a fall or other injury sustained because there
were not enough staff to cover the needs of patients on
that ward.

It is not unusual in whistleblowing for such a dilemma
to occur. A proactively accountable nurse confronts institutional constraints which hinder or block the nurse's
efforts to take action to remedy a situation of unsafe practice or potential abuse. Andersen (1990) identifies this
situation as causing 'moral distress', which is produced by
the cognitive dissonance of being unable even to gain
recognition of the problem, let alone to take action to
remedy or alleviate it. Thus the proactively accountable
nurse is left to climb the institutional ladder seeking redress
and validation of the situation. Unfortunately, the experience of whistleblowers has shown that even climbing up
this institutional ladder does not ensure that concerns will
be acted upon, validated or even listened to. The philosophy that what has existed as custom and practice for so
long within the institution without challenge must surely
be right not wrong — for it would have been challenged
before now — is fundamental to the institution's response
in dismissing the proactively accountable nurse's claims.
This, which Bernstein and Rozen (1989) have identified,
is known as 'dinosaur brain thinking'.

So Mary, upon her return to night duty and seeing that
nothing had changed from her discussion with the ward
sister, would continue to discuss and highlight her concerns over the low staffing on nights with the senior
sisters, the director of nursing services and even the general
manager of her hospital in an effort to reduce the cognitive

dissonance caused by the hospital's efforts to block Mary's attempts even to validate her own concerns and fears.

There comes a point at which the organisation can no longer tolerate the lone voice of a proactively accountable nurse. It is at this point that the system breaks down. Benign tolerance, with corrective sanctions to conform, is applied to adversarial factions where the integrity and ability of the proactively accountable nurse are being assaulted (Andersen, 1990). Slater (1990) refers to this stage as the 'toilet assumption', which is the 'notion that unwanted matter, unwanted difficulties, unwanted complexities and obstacles will disappear if they're removed from our immediate field of vision'. Thus, if Mary were to continue to pursue her concerns over the staffing levels on nights, she might well find that she has been moved to either another shift, another ward or even another area within the hospital to minimise her contact with those to whom she has been voicing her concerns. The 'toilet assumption' is that if she cannot be seen, her concerns are not visible, hence they do not exist.

It is at this stage that the personal attacks on the individual can turn moral distress into 'moral outrage'. Moral outrage (Andersen, 1990) 'occurs when a logical attempt to solve a moral problem results in denial of the problem and an assault on the nurse's integrity by those who have sacrificed their integrity and the welfare of patients to preserve the status quo of sub-marginal performance'. Some of the tactics used at this stage are isolating the whistleblower, making the whistleblower the problem rather than the issue, assigning the whistleblower impossible tasks with overwhelming obstacles, destabilising the whistleblower's support network, prosecuting her or him for obtaining information without consent or with breach of confidentiality and, finally, eliminating the job completely.

Thus for Mary, perhaps having been moved from nights

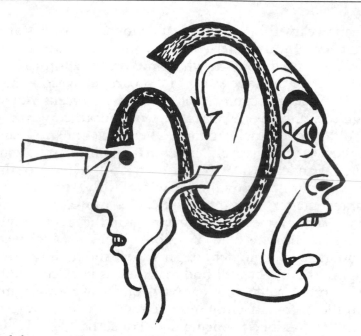

and her ward to, say, the intensive care unit, where her abilities would be questioned and her competence attacked, would produce within her the ingredients of moral outrage, e.g. emotional turbulence, distress, incredulity, indignation, anger and righteousness. At this stage, the individual seeks redress to maintain her or his own integrity and self-worth. It is no longer a question of solving the problem at hand but rather one of self-preservation, and once this stage is reached, it becomes very difficult to effect an equitable resolution within the existing internal framework of the organisation. Hence, the individual is left with going 'public' or with effecting external mechanisms to bring about change and justice on behalf of patients, as Graham Pink did, when in April 1990 after some eight months and 50 letters documenting 'a catalogue of neglect' (Turner, 1992), he allowed the *Guardian* to print a selection of his letters.

Loyalty and Fidelity

Hirschman (1970) has described the power of loyalty to the organisation as a deterrent to accountability, and Bok (1984) sees the act of the whistleblower as the ultimate betrayal because he or she is criticising from within and becomes, as described by Kiely and Kiely (1987), a traitor. These are very powerful words that have become real deterrents to whistleblowing. Mary certainly does not see herself as a traitor or as betraying the hospital. She clearly sees herself as a champion of her patients, ensuring that they receive the best possible care that she has been educated to provide. This dilemma is real, and it is one that pulls the potential whistleblower in many opposing directions, increasing the cognitive dissonance that he or she is already experiencing.

Fidelity is faithfulness and loyalty, and it is seen as the fundamental ethical principle from which all other principles are derived (Ramsay, 1970). It is certainly the basis for accountability (Catalano, 1991) and has had deep roots within nursing history since the days of Florence Nightingale. This excerpt, taken from *Practical Notes on Nursing Procedures* by Jessie Britten (Britten, 1966), illustrates the power of fidelity to nursing: 'The nurse must be loyally obedient to the medical staff, remembering that faith in the treatment goes a long way towards the patient's recovery'.

Not only is the nurse to be loyal to both the medical staff and nursing hierarchy, but implied in this statement is also the threat that loss of fidelity could result in patient harm through failure of the treatment. Is this underlying threat still present today? If a nurse voices concerns out of a sense of fidelity to her patients, and the Code of Professional Conduct (UKCC, 1992) states 'act always in such a manner as to promote and safeguard the interests and well being of patients and clients', could management be implying that by voicing these concerns, the nurse is actually harming her or his patient?

This was certainly the outcome of the case at Christie Hospital in February 1991, when one of the doctors went to the media about a patient with renal cell carcinoma who was denied treatment with interleukin 2, allegedly over cost (Walker, 1991). The subsequent enquiry concluded that the publicity was 'almost totally counterproductive'. Both staff and patients lost confidence in the hospital, several patients worried that they were not getting appropriate treatment because of cost, and fundraising become more difficult to secure because of the publicity (Smith, 1991).

Thus, the whistleblower experiences great conflict in having to choose between loyalty to the organisation and to the public. Yet from a different perspective, perhaps the whistleblower can still be seen to be loyal to both patients and the public at large, as well as to the organisation. In fact, the whistleblower might well be showing greater loyalty than that of the individual who does nothing in the face of neglect, abuse or immoral conduct. Fidelity involves acting in accordance with what one believes to be in the best interest of that individual or organisation. Thus, if an organisation is acting illegally or immorally, it is certainly not within that organisation's best interest to continue with such conduct. The employee who blows the whistle may therefore actually be demonstrating greater loyalty than the employee who simply ignores the immoral conduct, because the whistleblower is attempting to prevent the employer from engaging in self-destructive behaviour (Larmer, 1992).

But just as for accountability, fidelity can be conflicting. A nurse can have fidelity to her patient, yet this can conflict with her own sense of loyalty to herself through her own personal principles and values. Take, for example, the case of a patient who, even with both legs amputated owing to peripheral vascular disease, continues to smoke. The nurse may well value personal autonomy and freedom — the patient choosing to smoke — yet still hold true to the concept of non-maleficence: *primum non nocere*, 'above all do no harm'; passive smoking kills as well.

The same situation could be said to face Mary. She is being loyal to her patients by raising these concerns over the poor staffing levels on night duty, yet the hospital feels she is being disloyal to them as she is questioning and challenging their right as managers and budget holders to allocate scarce resources to the best of their ability with the concept of justice in mind. But, viewing this from Larmer's (1992) perspective, Mary could well be seen as being loyal to the hospital because in raising these concerns, she is highlighting potential areas of neglect that could give rise to very costly litigation. In that regard, Mary is protecting the organisation from self-harm and possible demise through closure due to financial constraints.

Justice

The above case history highlights one of the main dilemmas of whistleblowing, namely its unfairness. Here the nurse is risking all — her reputation, her integrity, her job, even her licence — to ensure that her patients receive that which they are entitled to receive, i.e. safe, competent and caring nursing. Yet in ensuring that they do receive what they are entitled to, she has suffered the distress of enduring condemnation, harassment, isolation and threats to her job security. Is this just?

Justice refers to the obligation to be fair to all people (Catalano, 1991), and it has three major areas of application: retributive justice, which is concerned with the punishment for wrongdoing; procedural justice, which focuses on the fairness of how things are done; and distributive justice, which is concerned with the allocation of resources, usually scarce resources (Fowler and Levine-Ariff, 1987). Within the multilayered concept of whistleblowing, all three types of justice come into play.

Retributive justice

By the time the whistleblower has reached the moral outrage stage, as described by Andersen (1990), retributive justice is high on the agenda. It becomes a moral imperative that those who have created the injustice for others feel the hand of justice on their own shoulder. So for Mary, after voicing her concerns and then being moved to another clinical area (intensive care) in which she did not have the skills and knowledge to perform, and then having been suspended over failure to perform an arterial blood gas analysis on a patient after extubation by the anaesthetist (a skill that Mary was not trained or competent in), it becomes vital that her self-respect is upheld by reporting the ward sister and others to the UKCC for abuse of their management position. In doing so, Mary is seeking retribution for the moral injustices she has endured.

Currently within law, there is very little protection for the potential whistleblower, unlike in the USA where there are several federal and state laws that give some protection (Government Accountability Project, 1989). Currently, a number of American whistleblowers are exercising retributive justice through *qui tam* lawsuits. *Qui tam* stands for *qui tam pro domino rege quam pro se ipso in hac parte sequitur*: 'He who sues on behalf of our Lord the King as well as for himself' (Bird, 1983). In other words, these are lawsuits brought on behalf of the government by the whistleblower, who, if successful, retains a percentage

of the judgement, in some cases making the whistleblower
a very wealthy individual (Vogel, 1991).

Procedural justice

At the moment, though, most whistleblowers in this
country are only able to seek redress through procedural
justice, i.e. industrial tribunals for wrongful dismissal. Procedural justice deals with the fairness of actions and procedures, not the rights or wrongs of a particular problem or
issue which led to the action or procedure occurring.
Thus, in Mary's case, should her suspension lead to dismissal, she would be able to seek redress through an industrial tribunal. The tribunal is not able to make a judgement
on the original problem of low staffing levels on nights; it
can only review the circumstances in which Mary was
dismissed and pass judgement on that procedure.

However, a favourable hearing does not always mean
reinstatement, as in the case of student nurse Ken Callanan.
In his case, *Callanan v. Surrey Area Health Authority*
(February 5 1980, COIT, 994/36), the tribunal found in
his favour, but it could not force the health authority to
reinstate him, nor was it able to make any judgement on
his original complaint of patient abuse (Beardshaw, 1981;
McHale, 1992).

More recently, in the case of Helen Zeitlin, the Sec-
retary of State for Health, Virginia Bottomley, ordered
that she be reinstated after a Department of Health hearing
(Greene and Cooper, 1992; Meek, 1992; Snell, 1992).
However, as with other cases of procedural justice, Dr
Zeitlin's original concerns about the nurse staffing levels
at the hospital have not been addressed. If the draft guidelines on whistleblowing, *Freedom of Speech for NHS Staff*
(DoH, 1992), are accepted, Dr Zeitlin's case will undoubt-
edly be the last hearing the Department of Health will
hold under the current appeals system. Under these new

draft guidelines, members of staff are only able to appeal
as far up as the chairman of the health authority or trust,
and no longer to the Department of Health. This, in
effect, is restricting procedural justice, for even in feudal
times, a serf was able to appeal to the lord of the manor!

Distributive justice

The final form of justice, distributive justice, refers to
fairness in the distribution of scarce resources, and, as the
RCN (1992) has highlighted, lack of resources has been a
recurrent theme in the letters it has received on whistleblowing. Within distributive justice, scarce resources are
usually allocated on one of the following criteria: effort/
merit, societal contribution, equal shares for each person,
according to need, or similar treatment for similar cases
(Fowler and Levine-Ariff, 1987).

Distributive justice has a large part to play in today's
health care settings, so it should not be surprising that it
will feature as an underlying theme in whistleblowing. For
Mary, the issue of lack of staff on nights has a very personal
effect as she has to meet the needs of all 31 of her patients
with the help of just one other nurse. From Mary's perspective, it feels to her that the distribution of staff nurses
on night duty is unfair. There were probably not enough
staff to meet all the needs of patients anyway, but at what
point does one draw the line? Who actually makes the
decision of which ward will or will not get the extra staff?
It certainly was not Mary, and repeatedly, for over three
weeks, she had been struggling to cope with the help that
she had.

But if Mary had carefully thought back or had kept
records and documented the care needs over the last three
weeks, would she honestly have admitted that there might
perhaps have been two or three hours once or twice a
week where things were not too bad? For a while, maybe

all the patients appeared to be sleeping, no-one was calling for the commode or bedpan, and no-one's drip needed changing or medication needed taking. At those times, when Mary could just relax and sit quietly at the desk, would she honestly have thought to have called up the night sister and say that as they were quiet for now, could she or the auxiliary offer some help to another ward? Somehow, human nature does not seem to work like that. It would only be natural for both Mary and the auxiliary to relax and rest for those few hours, and that would not be wrong.

However, what this does point out, though, are two fundamental problems with distributive justice, namely communication and truth-telling. Unless there are strong communication links between the various components of an organisation, it is very difficult for one part of the organisation to realise what is going on in another. This can work to both the advantage and disadvantage of the individual. Thus, when times are rich and plentiful, it is only natural to retain the bounty for oneself and one's patients. However, when times are lean and thin, it is only natural to scream for help. Unfortunately, there is very often not enough extra to go round because not everyone is being honest over what they currently have. How many times has the admission clerk telephoned for a bed check, only for the nurse to forget that 'Oh yes, I did discharge the patient in bay 2', because three of her four staff were at supper and she just could not cope with an admission at that moment? That nurse does not have the ability at that time to stop and think of the chain reaction that is caused by failing to disclose the bed.

Another factor in distributive justice is the nurse's ability to soldier on through insurmountable odds which slowly appear to become the norm and not the exception. Some nurses never or very rarely complain, while others state their case effectively and seem to obtain extra help. Again, this goes back to communication and the nurse's ability to assess and prioritise her patients' needs and ask for appropriate assistance. However, from Mary's perspective, it feels like never having had any help. Yes, the night sister did promise to send some relief for supper once or twice. What happened when that relief did not materialise? Did Mary shrug her shoulders saying, 'Well I didn't need the help anyway, what's one hour's help to me?' Or did she telephone the night sister asking where the reinforcement was? Perhaps in remaining silent, Mary gave the night sister the impression that she was managing effectively without help.

Distributive justice also works from the patient's perspective. There are physically only so many hospital beds — not an infinite number. Thus, when patients require hospitalisation, distributive justice comes into play allocating beds to those who need them most urgently, hence the ever-growing waiting lists for 'cold' surgery. But what about the patient who needs to have, for instance, coronary artery graft surgery, the man with a family of three small children who, through a familial tendency to hyperlipidaemia, has three blocked coronary arteries and now cannot have his life-saving surgery because a 19-year-old who stole a car, raced it recklessly at high speed and ran it straight into a tree, has just taken the last intensive care bed? Is that just?

So, has Mary assumed that all 31 of her patients have an equal right to their hospital bed? What about the 82-year-old widow and the 76-year-old man, both of whom need some attention and caring, but who have no medical problems that require hospitalisation? Their nursing needs revolve around providing nourishment and companionship. Yet the day staff are very reluctant to discharge them home as both live alone and neither has any support. Social services are involved and are desperately seeking out sheltered accommodation for them, but there are just not enough places to meet all the needs of the aging population. Hence, they remain in hospital with nowhere to go at the moment. Is that just?

When the individual begins to examine the situation in terms of distributive justice, it suddenly does not seem clear cut. Would Mary want these two elderly individuals to be discharged with no support, just so the workload on nights could be adequately covered by herself and the auxiliary? Would she then be prepared to let admissions know that she had two beds vacant, knowing full well that they soon would be filled with perhaps even sicker patients requiring more of her time? Is Mary being honest with her patients, the hospital, her manager and, more importantly, herself?

Truth or Veracity

Veracity, the obligation not only to tell the truth but also not to lie or deceive others, is fundamental as a concept to whistleblowing. The obligation of veracity is the foundation for respect, trust and loyalty between ourselves, our patients and our employers (Rumbold, 1986; Beauchamp and Childress, 1989). To tell the truth means that one tells the facts as one knows or comes to understand them — and herein lies the flaw. Truth then depends on an individual's perception of the facts, and, in some cases, two individuals may have opposing perceptions of any given set of facts.

In Mary's case, the real facts of the matter regarding the staffing levels on nights are that even though there are vacancies due to staff leaving, the hospital's budget is now overdrawn. Thus, there are no monies available to pay for any further nurses' salaries. Mary is unaware of the hospital's financial situation and can only perceive that there are vacancies that are not being filled. Management, on the other hand, not wanting to hear of the risks of further financial loss due to litigation because of low staffing, can only state that additional nurses are not needed. Is management deceiving Mary by not stating the real reason for not employing additional nurses – not that nurses are not needed, but that there is no money to pay for their salaries? But is that strictly true? What about the money that has been earmarked to refurbish the main reception area? Has Mary been told about that? More than likely not. So is this deception?

But to return to Mary's discussion with the ward sister. Here the sister accused Mary of not coping and not being able to prioritise her time. Is this the truth? To judge from Mary's reaction of anger and hurt at the accusation, it appears to be untrue. So, what are the facts on which the ward sister is basing her statement? Quite clearly, Mary is saying that she is having difficulty in coping on night duty with only one auxiliary. However, what sister knows but Mary does not is that Mary is the only staff nurse to complain about this situation. Even when asked, the other staff nurses state that they are not having any difficulties. And what neither Mary nor the ward sister knows, but the auxiliary does, is that Mary is the only staff nurse who actually goes on a one-hourly ward round every night, and if she sees any patient awake, she will go and tend to them. The other staff nurses do a ward round only three times a night, mostly just before the night sister appears to ensure that everything is quiet and in order. No wonder they can cope. Again, the auxiliary is holding on to a fact that neither of the other participants in this scenario has access to. Who is deceiving whom?

'Groupthink'

This type of situation can often lead to what Orwell spoke of as 'doublethink' and Janis (1982) as 'groupthink'. In this, group cohesiveness is so strong that any critical thinking or questioning of group norms, attitudes or behaviours tends to be regarded as deviance, even if it comes from within the group. Thus 'groupthink refers to a deterioration of mental efficiency, reality testing, and moral judgment that results from in-group pressures' (Janis, 1982). Groupthink tends to occur in situations where there is a high stress level from external threats of loss, along with a low hope of finding any solution other than the one put forward by the leader of the group. Could this be describing the National Health Service today?

Groupthink, coupled with Slater's (1990) operationalisation of the 'toilet assumption', certainly sets the stage for the behaviour that leads to what Andersen (1990) describes as 'moral distress' leading to 'moral outrage' of the whistleblower.

Conclusion

Uncovering all these layers of whistleblowing by examining the four ethical concepts of accountability, fidelity, justice and veracity can certainly enrich and hopefully enlighten any individual facing a similar situation and contemplating whistleblowing. The decisions are not easy, nor are they simple. Whistleblowing is a very complex concept with no absolutely correct solution. In what appears to be even the clearest of cases, there can always be another perspective.

Mary, the staff nurse whose case was used in this chapter, is in a situation where, owing to lack of resources, there are not enough night staff to cover the needs of patients on her particular ward. With only these facts available to her, Mary made the decision to raise this as a legitimate concern with her ward sister, who, for undisclosed reasons, chose to denigrate Mary for expressing these problems.

Had Mary thought out the consequences of her decision? How could Mary have enhanced her arguments at this stage of the situation? What else could Mary have done or said that would have persuaded the ward sister of the urgency of this situation?

Mary could have left the situation as it was, but being the proactive, accountable nurse that she is, and feeling it was her duty, she decided to pursue the matter when she returned to duty after her seven days off. Had Mary thought out the consequences of continuing this action? How could Mary have found out more information about this situation? Who else could she have turned to for advice?

The hospital management, unable to tolerate Mary's continued expressions of concern, chose to move her to another clinical area where she had no expertise or experience. Did they think out the consequences of their action? Could Mary have averted this action on the part of management? How could Mary now perform her duty to her patients on the acute medical ward when she was allocated to the intensive care unit? What becomes of her duty now? Had Mary thought out the consequences of accepting this new duty? Could Mary have foreseen that she would be asked, in this new clinical area, to perform skills that she had no experience of? Could Mary have averted the situation that resulted in her suspension? Who could Mary have turned to for advice? Did Mary know the procedure for filing a grievance, or the correct disciplinary procedure within her hospital and the NHS? Should Mary have been asking herself these and similar questions all along?

Despite the fact that there are no easy answers to the question of whether or not to blow the whistle on a situation, there are several common-sense precautions that can be taken which have been suggested by many sources (Beardshaw, 1981; Feliu, 1983; Clay, 1987; Kiely and Kiely,

1987; Government Accountability Project, 1989; Jackson, 1989; Andersen, 1990). These are:

- Before you blow the whistle, talk to your family and friends about the implication and consequences of this action. It will have a major impact on not only your own personal life but also that of your family and maybe even your friends. It could be that, with the additional information or an alternative perspective which either your family or friends can provide, an alternative to whistleblowing might be suggested.
- Aim to build up a network of support within the organisation. Start discussing the situation with other peers and co-workers. Have they perceived the same situation? Do they have additional information? Try to build some group cohesiveness about this situation. Do they feel the same as you?
- Depending on the circumstances of the situation, consider and use all the internal mechanisms for resolution before going 'outside', and make certain that you are aware of what these internal mechanisms are. If possible, rely on your network of support to cushion the impact of your disclosures. It is far more effective for a group to see the manager than just one individual, so let group dynamics work in your favour.
- Be respectful and treat all members of staff as you would wish to be treated. It becomes much harder to harass an individual who is 'such a nice person'. Be mindful of the effect that any action will be having on the other staff of the organisation as well. Some may not go along with the tactics of management; thus, your demeanour could have a positive effect on these individuals.
- Above all else, make certain that you have documented everything. It is very important that you

have a clear record of the events as they happen. Keep a diary not only of the events and the people involved but also of your feelings at the time. For significant happenings, it is wise to write 'Memoranda for the Record' as soon as possible after the event. Write out the situation as clearly and descriptively as you can remember, then sign and date it, having, if possible, someone to witness your signature. Then post it to yourself in a sealed envelope. Do not open it until it is required; its postmark will prove that it was written at the time of the event and not months later.

- Ensure that you have made copies of all relevant documents prior to disclosure, because, depending on the nature of the situation, access to records could be denied.
- Finally, make certain that you have discussed the situation with either your trade union, your professional representative or another specialist at the earliest possible stage. Their advice could be decisive. Do not attempt to go it alone without support or advice.

References

Andersen S (1990) Patient advocacy and whistle-blowing in nursing: help for the helpers. *Nursing Forum*, 25 (3): pp. 5–13.

Batey M and Lewis F (1982) Clarifying autonomy and accountability in nursing service: part 2. *The Journal of Nursing Administration*, 12 (10): pp. 10–15.

Beardshaw V (1981) *Conscientious Objectors at Work: Mental Hospital Nurses — A Case Study*. London: Social Audit.

Beauchamp T and Childress J (1989) *Principles of Biomedical Ethics* (3rd edn.). Oxford: Oxford University Press.

Bernstein A and Rozen S (1989) *Dinosaur Brains: Dealing with all those Impossible People at Work.* New York: John Wiley and Sons.

Bird R (1983) *Osborn's Concise Law Dictionary* (7th edn.). London: Sweet and Maxwell.

Boisjoly R, Curtis E and Mellican E (1989) Roger Boisjoly and the Challenger disaster: the ethical dimension. *Journal of Business Ethics*, 8 (4): pp. 217–30.

Bok S (1980) Whistleblowing and Professional Responsibility. *New York University Education Quarterly*, 10: pp. 2–10.

Bok S (1984) *Secrets: On the Ethics of Concealment and Revelation.* Oxford: Oxford University Press.

Britten J (1966) *Practical Notes on Nursing Procedures* (5th edn.). London: E and S Livingstone, Ltd.

Catalano J (1991) *Ethical and Legal Aspects of Nursing: A Study and Learning Tool.* Philadelphia: Springhouse Corporation.

Clay T (1987) *Nurses, Power and Politics.* London: Heinemann Nursing.

DoH (1992) *Freedom of Speech for NHS Staff — Draft Guidance,* 16 October 1992, 92/331. London: Department of Health.

Feliu A (1983) Thinking of blowing the whistle? *American Journal of Nursing,* 83 (11): pp. 1541–2.

Fiesta J (1990) Whistleblowers: heroes or stool pigeons? *Nursing Management,* 21 (6): pp. 16–17.

Fitzgerald K (1990) Engineering careers — whistle-blowing: not always a losing game. *IEEE Spectrum,* 27 (12): pp. 49–52.

Florman S (1989) Beyond whistleblowing. *Technology Review,* 92 (5): pp. 20, 76.

Fowler M and Levine-Ariff J (1987) *Ethics at the Bedside: A Source Book for the Critical Care Nurse.* Philadelphia: J B Lippincott.

Fraser A (1971) *Robin Hood.* London: Sidgwick and Jackson.

Government Accountability Project (1989) *Courage Without Martyrdom: A Survival Guide for Whistleblowers.* Washington, DC: Project on Government Procurement.

Greene D and Cooper J (1992) Whistle blowers. *BMJ,* 305: pp. 1343–4.

Hirschman A (1970) *Exit, Voice, and Loyalty.* Cambridge, Mass: Harvard University Press.

Jackson C (1989) Nothing to lose by speaking out. *Health Visitor*, 62: p. 191.

Janis I (1982) *Groupthink* (2nd edn.). Boston: Houghton Mifflin.

Jos P (1991) The nature and limits of the whistleblower's contribution to administrative responsibility. *American Review of Public Administration*, 21 (2): pp. 105–18.

Kiely M and Kiely D (1987) Whistleblowing: disclosure and its consequences for the professional nurse and management. *Nursing Management*, 18 (5): pp. 41–5.

Larmer R (1992) Whistleblowing and employee loyalty. *Journal of Business Ethics*, 11 (2): pp. 125–8.

McHale J (1992) Whistleblowing in the NHS. *The Journal of Social Welfare & Family Law*, no. 5: pp. 363–71.

Mason P (1992) Big rise in cases of managers abusing their authority. *Nursing Times*, 88 (38): p. 9.

Meek C (1992) Silencing the whistleblowers. *BMA New Review*, December: p. 17.

Ramsey P (1970) *The Patient as Person*. New Haven, Conn.: Yale University Press.

Royal College of Nursing (1992) *Whistleblow — Nurses Speak Out: A Report on the Work of the RCN Whistleblow Scheme*. London: RCN.

Rumbold G (1986) *Ethics in Nursing Practice*. London: Baillière Tindall.

Slater P (ed.) (1990) *The Pursuit of Loneliness: American Culture at Breaking Point* (3rd edn.). Boston: Beacon Press.

Smith R (1991) Christie Hospital reports on interleukin 2 controversy. *BMJ*, 302: p. 1041.

Snell J (1992) Whistle-blowing doctor to get job back. *Nursing Times*, 88 (46): p. 9.

Turner T (1992) The indomitable Mr. Pink. *Nursing Times*, 88 (24): pp. 26–9.

UKCC (1992) *Code of Professional Conduct* (3rd edn.). London: UKCC.

Vogel R (1991) Deterrent effects of whistleblower lawsuits justify false claims act. *Aviation Week & Space Technology*, 135 (18): pp. 73–4.

Walker A (1991) Interleukin 2 denied on grounds of cost. *BMJ*, 302: pp. 372–3.

Further Reading

Andersen S (1990) Patient advocacy and whistle-blowing in nursing: help for the helpers. *Nursing Forum*, 25 (3): pp. 5–13.
This article, written by a Canadian nurse educator, aims to empower student nurses by helping to describe the phenomenon of whistleblowing. She identifies two potential stages that an individual could experience during this process, namely moral distress and moral outrage. This approach is quite useful in enabling the individual to validate her or his own feelings during this process. There are a few case studies briefly described and the article ends with recommendations for future practice and research.

Beardshaw V (1981) *Conscientious Objectors at Work: Mental Hospital Nurses   A Case Study.* London: Social Audit.
This book is filled with good case material taken from real situations in the field of mental health nursing. It also describes the results of a survey of both student nurses and nurse educators on the question of whistleblowing. It portrays whistleblowing systematically and in a very realistic light and highlights some of the very real and dangerous pitfalls that can befall a whistleblower.

Bok S (1980) *Lying: Moral Choice in Public and Private Life.* London: Quartet.

Bok S (1984) *Secrets: On the Ethics of Concealment and Revelation.* Oxford: Oxford University Press.
Both these books by Sissela Bok have contributed greatly to the discussion and understanding of the conditions that prevail within a whistleblowing scenario. Knowledge is power, and an understanding of both of these elements within whistleblowing certainly helps the individual to come to understand what might be happening in these situations.

McHale J (1992) Whistleblowing in the NHS. *The Journal of Social Welfare & Family Law*, no. 5: pp. 363–71.
This article examines the legal aspects of whistleblowing, focusing on both American and English cases. It examines the consequences of disclosure and highlights the role of

industrial tribunals and the courts, offering some suggestions for reform of the law in the UK.

Menzies-Lyth I (1988) The functioning of social systems as a defence against anxiety (1959, 1961, 1970). *Containing Anxiety in Institutions: Selected Essays, vol. 1.* London: Free Association Books.

A very good resource for understanding the hidden dynamics present in whistleblowing situations within the institutional setting of hospitals. Menzies-Lyth examined the social defence system of a large London teaching hospital and concluded that this represented the institutionalisation of very primitive psychic defence mechanisms which facilitated the evasion of anxiety but did little to help reduce or modify its presence.

Plant R (1987) *Managing Change and Making it Stick.* London: Fontana/Collins.

The process of change very often uncovers situations that result in whistleblowing. This little book is excellent in describing the processes of change and how they affect the individual. As the author states, there are no answers in this book, but it certainly will help to formulate the right questions to ask.

Wilson D (1992) *A Strategy of Change: Concepts and Controversies in the Management of Change*, London: Routledge.

This book examines the area of organisational change and survival in the 1990s. It is a good description of the new management culture and helps to give a broad understanding through critical analysis of these changes. It has a detailed and excellent reference list at the end and draws on material from a wide range of topics.

Winfield M (1990) *Minding Your Own Business.* London: Social Audit.

This book examines the process of whistleblowing in British business and reports on the result of a survey of 53 companies, examining how these businesses regulate themselves. It is full of good example and cases, highlights relevant laws that could affect the whistleblower, and gives a detailed account of the process of whistleblowing. There is a good reference list at the end.

CHAPTER 4

Competing Values

Maureen Eby

Nurses are often — too often perhaps — in situations where their values conflict with those of their patients, medical colleagues and employers. What criteria do they use to resolve the conflict?

The author illustrates this dilemma with a personal example. Had she known then what she has detailed in this chapter, she might not have had the pain which this episode caused her. The reader is presented with different theories of decision-making, which are based on the idea of cognitive dissonance and seeking consistency. Detailing such theories should stimulate nurses to turn them into practice for their own advantage and that of their patients and colleagues.

In the course of nursing, situations will arise in which values compete against one another. This can occur on both personal and interpersonal levels as well as at an organisational level. As individuals, we each hold our own set of personal values and principles that govern our lives. For the most part, these values are usually compatible with other values found within society and, on the whole, conflicts tend to be rare. However, there are times when individual values will come into conflict with those of other individuals and/or society. The following case history illustrates some of these conflicts.

A Case History

It was my first ward as a newly qualified staff nurse, a 44-bed neurosurgical ward on which the patients ranged from those

awaiting neurosurgery for their newly diagnosed tumours to
those having chemotherapy and radiation therapy or being
readmitted in the advanced terminal stages of malignant brain
tumours. Among the 11 patients for whom I had responsibility as
their primary nurse was Mrs Minnosa, who had been on the unit
for six weeks.

Mrs Minnosa, widowed with one son, had been admitted with
headaches, seizures and left-sided hemiparesis. Diagnostic
tests had revealed a meningioma, well-encapsulated and very
amenable to surgical intervention. Her seizures were currently
under control with medication, but her hemiparesis and
incontinence were quite distressing to her. Nevertheless, her
mind was still sharp and she was very vocal in stating her needs
and opinions. 'No', she kept stating repeatedly, 'I will not have
any surgery . . . no one is cutting into my head!' She constantly
upheld this view, and, despite discussions with her son and
the neurosurgeon, Mrs Minnosa would not consent to surgery.

Mrs Minnosa's insistence that she would not have this
surgery confounded and dismayed me. Could she not
understand that her brain tumour was not malignant? The
neurosurgeon kept repeating to her and her son that this
tumour was not cancer and that, when it had been surgically
removed, Mrs Minnosa's distressing symptoms would disappear.
As a nurse, I had no difficulty in understanding what the
neurosurgeon was saying, or in believing it, but Mrs Minnosa
kept insisting that the neurosurgeon was tricking her into surgery
as 'he just wants to cut my mind out'.

Mrs Minnosa's son spent weeks trying to convince his mother
to have the surgery, and all I could see was his mounting
frustration as she continued to refuse. Even though she
appeared to understand that the tumour was not cancerous,
she had a real fear that in cutting out the tumour, the
neurosurgeon would also be cutting out her 'mind'. No amount
of reassurance that her mind would not be affected would alter
this fact, and it now seemed that Mrs Minnosa was adamant
and, even with an increase in her symptoms, would still not
consent to surgery.

After eight weeks, the neurosurgeon and the hospital, with her son's permission, made an application to the courts to obtain consent on the grounds of diminished competence. The neurosurgeon stated that the meningioma was impairing Mrs Minnosa's judgement, and, on those grounds, consent was given for the neurosurgeon to operate, despite the fact that Mrs Minnosa was still verbally insisting that she would not have the surgery. Even when told that consent had been given through the courts, Mrs Minnosa was still insistent that she would not go to theatre.

By now, as Mrs Minnosa's nurse, I was really torn. I could see her right to autonomy, to make judgements and decisions on her own, but was the neurosurgeon right in his belief that her judgement was impaired by the meningioma? In all other respects, Mrs Minnosa was able to make other decisions in her life: when to get out of bed, what to wear, what to order from the dinner menu and when to have her morning wash or wash her hair. She was able to read the newspaper (though this was getting progressively more difficult for her) and watch television, and she was very forthright in stating her opinions on the events of the day. This was Mrs Minnosa's life, and she had a right to decide her future for herself, but somehow I also had this overriding feeling that it was not just Mrs Minnosa's right for autonomy that was at issue, for I, too, as her nurse felt that I had a right to do good for her.

My knowledge of Mrs Minnosa's meningioma enabled me to understand the necessity of surgery, and I knew that it would remove her distressing symptoms. The meningioma was clearly identifiable on the CAT scan, and I could not understand her reasoning that the neurosurgeon was tricking her into surgery to remove her mind. Surgery was going to benefit Mrs Minnosa, not harm her further. This was my firm belief even after spending weeks of trying to understand Mrs Minnosa's reasoning. To me the principle of beneficence was equally as strong as Mrs Minnosa's right to autonomy and personal freedom in this situation. Thus, the value of beneficence which was embedded in my own personal sense of my worth and value as a nurse

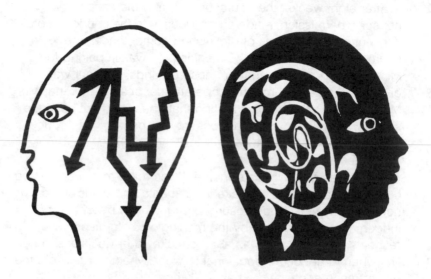

was in direct conflict with Mrs Minnosa's equally embedded
personal right to autonomy; in other words, what had
developed was a situation of competing values.

Competing Values

An ethical issue is one in which two or more values or
principles are present but a conflict has not occurred
between them. However, an ethical problem is when there
is a conflict between these competing values and principles
(Purtilo, 1993).

Ethical problems can either cause distress or create
dilemmas. Ethical distress is caused when barriers prevent
the right course of action from occurring, while an ethical
dilemma occurs when there is a choice between two
equally right or wrong courses of action, in which either
choice will result in compromise of the values or principles

involved (Benjamin and Curtis, 1986; Thompson, Melia and Boyd, 1988; Tschudin, 1992; Purtilo, 1993). An ethical dilemma, as stipulated by Curtin (1982) in Marquis and Huston (1992), also requires three other conditions: that the problem cannot be solved using empirical data alone, that it must be so perplexing that it is very difficult to identify the facts needed to make the decision, and finally that the results of the decision will have far-reaching effects beyond just the immediate decision itself. In the case of Mrs Minnosa, the dilemma caused not only ethical distress, because Mrs Minnosa's reasoning created a barrier, but also a dilemma owing to the conflicting choice of whether or not to operate.

However, ethical dilemmas can be created over personal competing values as well as competing values between oneself and the organisation. On a personal level, the principle of autonomy or individual freedom can often conflict with the principle of non-maleficence, i.e. to do no harm. This is usually seen as a conflict over personal lifestyles (such as between one's beliefs and behaviours over smoking or drinking alcohol), but dilemmas can also occur between other values and principles, such as truth-telling and non-maleficence. For example, if you are aware your friend is going out with an individual you know to be married, do you tell her, realising that it might cause her great pain, or do you not tell her and risk losing the friendship if she finds out later that you knew?

At an organisational level, you may well find yourself having to decide between upholding the Code of Professional Conduct (UKCC, 1992) or risk losing your job as a nurse and/or your registration to practise in a situation where the organisation has compromised on quality and service due to the financial constraints imposed through governmental reforms. It is the tensions that these conflicts create that very often drive the nurse to seek out answers.

Cognitive Dissonance

This state of tension is known as cognitive dissonance and occurs when an individual holds inconsistent beliefs and attitudes or when an individual's behaviour does not match his or her attitudes and belief system. This tension is experienced as increasing discomfort, described as a negative drive force that motivates the individual to reduce the dissonance by seeking out ways to achieve consistency in attitudes, beliefs and/or behaviours (Festinger, 1964; Lippa, 1990).

Underlying this notion of cognitive dissonance is the theory of cognitive consistency, which states as its basic premise that all humans strive to be consistent in their beliefs, attitudes and behaviours, and it is the inconsistency of beliefs, attitudes and behaviours that acts as an irritant or stimulus to modify or change this inconsistency so that consistency is again achieved (Atkinson et al, 1990). Cognitive consistency, or 'balance theory', was developed by Heider in the late 1940s, and it relies on two fundamental assumptions: firstly, that individuals are aware of their attitudes and beliefs, and secondly, that individuals are motivated to keep these attitudes and beliefs consistent. However, even though individuals are driven to remain consistent in their attitudes, beliefs and behaviours, it does not necessarily mean that individuals are rational or even logical in achieving this consistency (Deaux, Dane and Wrightsman, 1993).

Cognitive dissonance theory as developed by Festinger in the late 1950s originally stated that dissonance occurred whenever an individual had inconsistent beliefs, attitudes and/or behaviours, but was later refined by others to state that for dissonance to be maximised, individuals must feel that their inconsistent attitudes and/or behaviours were freely chosen and were their own personal responsibility, that they were firmly committed and irrevocable, and that they had important consequences for others (Lippa, 1990). This feeling of dissonance that is created by simultaneously having inconsistent attitudes, beliefs and/ or behaviours becomes a powerful motivating force simi- lar — in the words of Festinger (1964) — to hunger and thirst.

Just as the individual is driven to seek out food and water when hungry and thirsty, so it is with cognitive dissonance: the person is driven to reduce these negative, irritable and uncomfortable feelings. Thus, the greater the feeling of dissonance, the stronger the motivation to reduce it to a state of consistency (Brown, 1965; Heckhausen and Weiner, 1972; and Radford and Govier, 1980). In order to achieve this consistency of attitudes, beliefs and/or behaviours, Festinger suggests that the individual experien- cing dissonance will either discount or ignore the incon- sistent information, reinterpret or reappraise the inconsistent information to bring it in line with consist- ency, or actively seek out additional supporting infor- mation to reinforce the currently held attitudes and belief systems (Beloff, 1973; Radford and Govier, 1980).

As with hunger and thirst, the drive to seek out consist- ency is not always a deliberate, well thought out and conscious process, but one that is often arrived at in haste and through the desire to achieve the relief of uncomfort- able feelings. It is similar to the ravenous individual who quickly gulps down food, often developing heartburn in the process, just to feel the satisfaction of relief from those uncomfortable feelings of hunger.

Brehm (1956) in Radford and Govier (1980), applying Festinger's theory to decision-making, discovered that dissonance is aroused through having made a decision between two or more alternative courses of action; this he termed post-decisional dissonance. The effect of this dissonance is proportional to the importance of the decision to the individual, the attractiveness of the unchosen alternative, and the degree to which the alternative choices differ. Through his research, Brehm suggested that two ways of decreasing the dissonance created by this decision–making dilemma were to decrease the attractiveness of the unchosen alternative and to increase the attractiveness of the chosen alternative.

The application of cognitive dissonance theory

Considering the case history above, Mrs Minnosa's insistence that she would not consent to surgery both confounded and dismayed me. These feelings were my burgeoning awareness of experiencing dissonance. I was struggling to achieve a balance or consistency between my personal beliefs, as well as my beliefs and behaviour as a nurse, and Mrs Minnosa's behaviour. It was the dissonance, these uncomfortable feelings of bewilderment and anger, that drove me to keep on listening to Mrs Minnosa's reasoning in the hope that somewhere within her logic I could find a way of adapting my beliefs so that they would conform to her behaviour, or that by continuing to listen, I might be able to correct her misperceptions in order that her behaviour might change to meet my beliefs.

My feelings of dissonance were made even more acute by the fact that Mrs Minnosa's decision not to have surgery was freely chosen and was her own responsibility. It certainly was a committed choice and appeared irrevocable, and it would have consequences not only for her, probably by her death, but also for her son in the loss of his mother.

I was never able to resolve this dilemma. In all the weeks I spent with Mrs Minnosa, I was never able to see anything within her logical framework to which I could adapt my personal belief system so that it would match hers, nor could I find any way of overcoming her misperceptions of the neurosurgeon. It was only when the neurosurgeon obtained consent through the courts that I realised

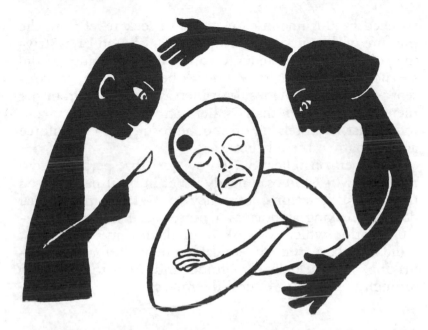

that I had failed Mrs Minnosa and that, in fact, despite her protests, she would be having this surgery.

That I no longer had any control in this situation increased my feelings of dissonance. However, as my dissonance increased, so did its impact as a motivational drive to reach consistency, for once the neurosurgeon had obtained consent, that began to reinforce my belief system that as a nurse I was there to do good (the principle of beneficence). I began to see signs in Mrs Minnosa that reinforced the beliefs of the neurosurgeon that Mrs Minnosa was not, in fact, competent to make this decision. So like the hungry person, I was grabbing at anything that would reduce the uncomfortable feelings of dissonance. Thus, several days later, Mrs Minnosa went down to theatre, protesting and yelling for help all the way, and, yes, I was able to accompany her.

Even though I felt helpless and frustrated for Mrs Minnosa, the dissonance within myself had been significantly

reduced by this unconscious drive to seek relief from the
pressure of the uncomfortable feelings. I found I was striv-
ing to achieve consistency through reinterpreting (as did
the neurosurgeon) Mrs Minnosa's behaviour not to consent to surgery as the result of increased pressure from her
meningioma rather than as her rational decision. I also
found that I was relying on the neurosurgeon to reinforce
and strengthen these beliefs.

However, on reflection, I now feel that perhaps I did
not meet Mrs Minnosa's needs as her nurse. I had allowed
the human drive for consistency to override my rational
decision-making abilities as a nurse, for I had no framework within which to work through this situation. What
I did not have was an ethical framework for decision-
making, which helps to guide and ease the traveller
through the maze of ethical dilemmas.

Ethical Decision-making Frameworks

Ethics, like nursing, is not a product, yet many nurses
approach the door of ethics with a shopping list of questions to which they want answers. Confronting the
dilemmas of nursing practice is no different from confronting the challenges of a patient's malodorous and suppurat-
ing pressure sore, yet nurses continue to feel that these
ethical dilemmas of practice are different and demand
concrete answers from the law and ethics. When these
answers are not forthcoming, the nurse's dissonance
increases.

If one alters one's perspective to thinking that ethics is
a process just like nursing is a process, the ethical dilemmas
that loom like a forbidding mountain suddenly become
less threatening and, hopefully, more manageable. Like the
nursing process, ethical decision-making is a process, and
once one applies a systematic framework to the dilemma,

choices become clearer, although the decision may still not be an easy one. There are many ethical decision-making frameworks available in medical and nursing ethics textbooks as well as in journal articles, most, although not all, using a nursing process framework of assessing, planning, implementing and evaluating.

In selecting a framework, one needs to think of its underlying assumptions and beliefs and compare these to one's own personal belief systems. Some of these frameworks may be cumbersome, others very easy to use, but either way one needs to select a framework that works well on a personal level.

The most frequently used framework revolves around a five-step process of:

- assess the situation;
- identify the ethical/moral problems;
- set ethical/moral goals and plan the action;
- implement the plan of action;
- evaluate the outcomes. (Johnstone, 1989)

The individual steps of this five-step process can be described as:

- gather the relevant information;
- identify the types of ethical problem;
- determine the ethics approach to be used;
- explore the practical alternatives;
- complete the action. (Purtilo, 1993)

Information-gathering

The first step of the decision-making process is similar to that of the nursing process in that it aims to collect all the relevant information about the situation creating the dilemma. In this step, one is seeking out facts, attitudes, beliefs and external factors. Sometimes, it helps to ask a series of questions at this stage to ensure that all the relevant facts and points of view have been identified. It also helps to reflect on the situation at different points in time to ensure that all possible factors have been thought of. Jonsen, Siegler and Winslade (1986, in Purtilo, 1993) suggest four major areas of information that may be useful to structure information-gathering:

- *Clinical indications* — such as the patient's condition, the prognosis, the treatment choices available and the outcomes for each treatment option.
- *Patient preferences* — which would include whether the patient was informed of all the available choices, whether the patient was competent to choose, and if not, why not, whether someone else could choose for the patient and, if so, who.
- *Quality of life issues* — looking at these from both the patient's and the health professional's perspective as well as seeing the effect of each treatment option on the patient's quality of life.
- *External factors* — which are very important but often overlooked in decision-making, for example what hospital policies there are that might affect this decision, whether there are any legal implications involved, whether resource allocation or rationing is a factor, and what the professional bodies or organisations have to say on this matter.

Identifying the problem

The second step of identifying the moral or ethical problems requires that the individual have some working knowledge of ethical principles, such as Thiroux's (1980, in Tschudin, 1992) five principles of the value of life, goodness or rightness, justice or fairness, truth-telling or honesty, and individual freedom, or Gillon's (1986, in

Tschudin, 1992) four principles of autonomy, justice, beneficence and non-maleficence.

However as Johnstone (1989) points out, it is useful at this stage to be very open minded, for it is possible that what appears to be a moral problem might instead actually be 'a problem of poor communication, misunderstanding, a misinterpretation of the facts, ignorance of the legal law or institutional policy or cultural unawareness'. Johnstone goes on further to describe some pitfalls and misconceptions which nurses encounter when identifying moral problems, namely moral unpreparedness, moral blindness, moral indifference, amoralism, moral complacency and moral fanaticism.

Identifying the problem is crucial, as it is in the nursing process, for if at this stage actual or potential problems are not identified or have been misdiagnosed, the subsequent steps of the process will be inadequate and incomplete.

Goals and actions

It is at this third step that ethical decision-making frameworks tend to differ, as can be seen from the two approaches above (Johnstone, 1989 and Purtilo, 1993). One is set in determining moral goals or planning an appropriate course of action, while the other concentrates on examining the identified problems from the dual perspective of utilitarianism and deontology. In this sense, the Purtilo (1993) framework forces the nurse to examine the identified problems in more detail from opposing ethical frameworks, and, as such, this step could also be seen as a framework within a framework.

Found within Candee and Puka's (1988) article on medical ethics are two frameworks that outline the steps of the moral reasoning process from this dual theoretical perspective; one outlines the utilitarian (teleological) approach and the other the deontological approach. Utili-

tarian theory aims to determine which course of action
will produce the greatest benefit over harm for all the
individuals involved in the situation, while the deontological approach examines the rights, duties and principles
involved in a dilemma and tries to determine which of
these takes precedence in the particular situation. Candee
and Puka's frameworks are outlined in Table 1.

Table 1 Steps in the moral reasoning process (adapted
from Candee and Puka, 1988)

Teleological approach	Deontological approach
• List the identified problems	• List the identified problems
• List the feasible alternatives	• List the feasible alternatives
• Predict the consequence (outcomes) for each of these alternatives	• Specify all the relevant rights, duties and principles
• Determine the probability of each of these outcomes occurring	• Establish the validity of these rights, duties and principles
• Prioritise these outcomes, specifying the basis for your prioritisation	• Determine the priorities and identify which takes precedence
• Determine the utility or benefit to harm ratio for each of these alternatives	• Choose a course of action
• Choose a course of action	

Thus in working through both of these frameworks, a
dual perspective can be generated that enables one to
examine the identified problem from alternative perspec-

tives. There are, however, other perspectives besides that of deontology/teleology, namely Frankena's (1973) theory of obligation, which examines the principles of beneficence and justice, Firth's (1970) ideal observer theory and Rawls' (1971) justice as fairness theory (all cited in Davis and Aroskar, 1983).

In Frankena's theory of obligation, the nurse should consider the alternatives of action from the basis of the principles of beneficence and justice being equal, while with Firth's ideal observer theory, the nurse should consider the alternatives of action from a disinterested, dispassionate, omniscient and consistent point of view. However, in Rawls' theory of justice as fairness, the nurse should consider the alternatives of action from the point of view of the least fortunate in society (Davis and Aroskar, 1983; Rumbold, 1986; Beauchamp and Childress, 1989; Bandman and Bandman, 1990). Thus, as can be seen, determining the ethical approach to be used is a very useful and enriching step in the process.

There are, however, some pitfalls to be aware of in working through this step of the process, namely fallacies in reasoning. By learning to identify and correct fallacies in reasoning, effective and justifiable decision-making can be facilitated. Some of the more common fallacies that nurses are exposed to are listed below (Bandman and Bandman, 1990):

- **the is–ought fallacy** argues that if a decision or policy is in effect for an individual then it ought to be in effect for everyone. So if Mr Smith is going to be resuscitated then everyone should be resuscitated.
- **appeal to force** consists of ensuring that another individual accepts your conclusions on the basis of force alone, such as 'If you don't take your medi-

cation, your heart will stop!' or 'If you don't have
this surgery, you will die!'

- **abuse of the person** consists of abusing the individual in the argument, such as 'You kept on resuscit-
  ating because of your own sense of morality . . . you
  can't accept defeat, can you!' or 'It's only because
  you're a Catholic that you won't look after that abor-
  tion patient!'

- **appeal to populace** argues that if everybody does
  it then it must be good, i.e. 'Everyone does overtime,
  so it must be good or important to do overtime' or
  'Drinking on duty at Christmas is acceptable because
  everyone drinks at Christmas.'

- **appeal to authority** is a common fallacy which
  entails individuals with appropriate authority pres-
  enting themselves as authorities outside their area of
  expertise, such as 'You are not going to like this, but
  I am going to get you out of bed. You will thank
  me for this later. It might be painful now but
  believe me I know the pain will only get worse if
  you don't walk.'

- **the slippery slope fallacy** is often used in arguments against active euthanasia. 'If we allow voluntary, active euthanasia for individuals at their own
  request, even with strict controls, then we're heading
  down the slippery slope of allowing the euthanasia
  of individuals with dementia, Alzheimer's, the handi-
  capped . . . where would it end?'

- **slothful induction** is the refusal to listen or think
  about any contradictory information which would
  refute your argument, such as the anti-abortionist
  who does not consider the woman's right to her own
  body or the pro-abortionist not including the rights
  of the fetus in their argument.

- **the fallacy of accident** is when an individual indis-
  criminately applies an ethical principle without regard

to individual circumstances or differences, such as the principle 'I will keep all confidences confidential', which can have disastrous consequences if a patient discloses to the nurse that he intends to kill his wife because he suspects she is 'cheating' on him.

- **the complex question** is a fallacy which asks a question, the answer of which is dependent on a previous question. 'Will you give up smoking and have this surgery because without this surgery you will die!'

This third step in the decision-making process is a vital one, for it is at this point that one comes to terms with the principles involved and really starts to challenge and examine one's own personal underlying belief systems at work in the dilemma. It is at this point that personal learning can occur.

Implementing the action plan

The fourth and fifth steps in the decision-making process tend to be universally similar in that a plan of action is identified or the practical alternatives are specified, based on the analysis of the problems conducted in the third step of the process. If more than one plan of action has already been worked out these should have been prioritised so that one preferred course of action is left, which is then implemented.

Evaluating the outcomes

Not all of these frameworks for decision-making add the step of evaluation, which is crucial in determining the strengths and weaknesses not only of the framework itself but also of one's assessment skills, reasoning ability and, finally, knowledge base. This step can also enhance learning, for it allows one to examine the relationship of the stated outcomes to the actual outcomes and assists with identifying alternatives for future decision-making.

Tschudin (1992) raises a number of important questions that should be asked at this stage, for instance: did the agreed decision solve the problem?; what was gained by the participants in this decision?; and how do the individuals involved in this decision feel about the problem now? As well as focusing on the problems and resolution, it is important to evaluate the problem-solving process used in terms of its future application, e.g. if one were faced with this decision again, would the same choice be made; or, has this made the process of ethical decision-making any easier in the future?

Variations on the Process Framework of Ethical Decision-Making

There are many other variations on this process framework for ethical decision-making. Tschudin (1992) describes another variation on this five-step process, namely Crisham's (1985) model which identifies the following steps and is remembered by the mnemonic MORAL:

M — 'Massage' the dilemma or explore the dilemma in all its complexities.
O — Outline the options.
R — Review the criteria or alternatives.
A — Act.
L — Look back, review or evaluate.

Brown, Kitson and McKnight (1992) also have a variation on the five-step process which redistributes the steps in a slightly different sequence, namely:

- Stage 1 — Appreciation of the situation.
- Stage 2 — Review of possible actions.

- Stage 3 — Selecting and applying principles.
- Stage 4 — Weighing practical considerations.
- Stage 5 — Decision.

Uustal (1990) describes a nine-step process, which in fact just expands step three into five separate steps:

1. Identify the problem.
2. State your values and ethical position related to the case, as well as those of the patient and other individuals involved in this situation.
3. Identify alternatives for resolving the dilemma.
4. Examine and categorise these choices.
5. Identify the possible consequences of each of the possible choices.
6. Prioritise the acceptable choices.
7. Develop your plan of action.
8. Implement this plan of action.
9. Evaluate the outcomes of this plan of action.

Finally, Pellegrino (1981) has devised a much simplified three-step process framework, which does not rely on an extensive ethical knowledge base but draws on the individual's common sense. Essentially, Pellegrino asks just three questions:

- **What is the problem?** — the assessment phase: can the problem be simply stated?; is there more than one problem involved?
- **What can be done?** — what are all the options available? What are the benefits and adverse effects of each of these options?
- **What should be done?** — what is best for the patient? What is important to the patient? What is right or wrong for the patient?

Again, this ethical framework does not have an evaluative phase, but as with the nursing process, evaluation should

be an ongoing process constantly feeding into the assessment phase of the process after the decision has been made
or the problem solved. This particular framework is very
simple and is deceptively easy to use; however, it does
require that one develops an awareness of moral and ethical
issues and does not become either morally unprepared,
blind or indifferent.

Complex Ethical Decision-making Frameworks

There are more complex ethical decision-making frameworks available for those who prefer a model or pathways
approach to decision-making. Two are found within the
realm of medical ethics and two within nursing ethics.

Seedhouse (1988, 1991, and Seedhouse and Lovett,
1992) has devised both an ethical grid and an algorithm
to aid in ethical decision-making. The grid is designed
in a grid boxed system made up of individual colours
representing the different layers involved in ethical
decision-making. As such, the grid incorporates a number
of ethical theories and concepts and is a precis to aid
the individual. The four coloured levels of the grid are
(Seedhouse and Lovett, 1992):

- Black — the level of practicality.
- Green — the level of consequences.
- Red — the level of duties.
- Blue — the basis of health care.

The algorithm was devised to be more systematic in its
approach to ethical decision-making and is constructed
from the individual components of the grid in a pathway
or decision-tree format. The algorithm is divided into four
quadrants based on the four layers of the grid, and the
individuals start in the quadrant which has the most
immediate relevance to them. Both the grid and the algor-

ithm require a systematic and logical approach to decision-making; however, they have been construed as being inflexible by some. Since they are systematic, both of these approaches allow for each ethical issue to be examined in detail, ensuring that all aspects of the dilemma have been explored.

Johnson (1990) has constructed a simplified pathway system (algorithm) that starts with the clinical situation and ends with an examination of the fallacies of reasoning. This framework is based on an examination of the ethical principles and the consequences involved in the ethical issue. This is an interesting and useful framework as it allows the individual first of all to identify whether, in fact, the issue arising from the clinical situation is an ethical issue or instead a technical problem, an emotional problem or a question of etiquette.

Once it has been determined that there is in fact an ethical issue, the individual moves through the decision tree to examine the components of the issue, i.e. aims, values, autonomy and truth, in the light of the general and specific ethical principles that interplay within this issue. This method of ethical decision-making parallels quite closely the clinical decision-making skills that doctors need to develop and, as such, it is seen as an extension to the logical and systematic way of approaching decision-making.

Husted and Husted (1991) have developed a simplified pathway which starts with the nurse–patient agreement and ends with a decision. Fundamental to this pathway is the nurse–patient interaction, which is based on agreement rather than deception or coercion. Fundamental to this nurse–patient agreement are the bioethical concepts of autonomy, freedom, veracity, privacy, beneficence and fidelity. Thus, each dilemma is analysed in terms of these six concepts in the light of the context of the situation and the knowledge involved. Despite its appearing to be a simplified pathway it is actually quite complicated in terms of its application and requires that one reads through the entire text really to understand how the pathway operates.

Finally, Greipp's (1992) model of ethical decision-making is based on general systems theory and the work of Leininger and her theory of transcultural caring (1978, in Greipp, 1992). Again, it appears to be quite a complicated model, with both the nurse and the client feeding into the decision-making process. The nurse has a fairly complicated framework to pass through, which examines the concepts of autonomy, beneficence, responsibility, accountability, knowledge, non-maleficence and justice as involved in the dilemma. Greipp stresses that the value of this model for the nurse 'lies in its diagrammatic structure which will keep the nurse focused and aware of the influence that psychosociocultural variables have on decision-making interactions' (Greipp, 1992).

Conclusion

As health care is changing due to governmental reforms, the state of the economy, the rise of long-term and chronic illnesses and the changing nature of nursing as a profession, ethical issues and problems will continue to emerge. Part of developing as a competent and caring nurse is the ability to adapt and thrive in the ever-changing environment of today's health service. Attempting to solve both clinical and ethical issues and problems without the aid of some sort of framework will only increase the frustration and dissonance that nurses are currently feeling, and, more importantly, it will force nurses to rely on the human drive for consistency to guide their decision-making rather than allow for the conscious, deliberate and systematic process of decision-making that is needed.

In the case of Mrs Minnosa above, no ethical framework was used to aid the decision-making process. To resolve the dilemma, the neurosurgeon went to court to obtain consent for surgery to remove Mrs Minnosa's meningioma. Unfortunately, from the nurse's perspective the dilemma had not been resolved, but rather the dissonance from a nursing point of view had been reduced through the human drive for consistency.

If an ethical framework had been used, what difference would that have made to the outcome? Perhaps, if I had consciously and systematically worked through an ethical framework with Mrs Minnosa, her son and the neurosurgeon, I might have found that my role as an advocate would have been more clearly identified and strengthened. Unfortunately, I was not able to reach that conclusion. In the end, Mrs Minnosa did have surgery to remove the meningioma, but as the meningioma had been exerting ever-increasing pressure on vital parts of her brain, the symptoms were not relieved by removing the tumour. Thus, Mrs Minnosa was partially correct in her beliefs. She still required medication to control her seizures and she still had residual hemiparesis and incontinence. Four weeks after her surgery, Mrs Minnosa was transferred to a nursing home as her son was unable to care for her due to her many physical problems.

References

Atkinson R, Atkinson R, Smith E, Bem D and Hilgard E (1990) *Introduction to Psychology* (10th edn.). New York: Harcourt Brace Jovanovich.

Bandman E and Bandman B (1990) *Nursing Ethics Through the Life Span* (2nd edn.). Englewood Cliffs, NJ: Prentice Hall.

Beauchamp T and Childress J (1989) *Principles of Biomedical Ethics* (3rd edn.). Oxford: Oxford University Press.

Beloff J (1973) *Psychological Sciences: A Review of Modern Psychology.* London: Crosby Lockwood Staples.

Benjamin M and Curtis J (1986) *Ethics in Nursing* (2nd edn.). Oxford: Oxford University Press.

Brown J, Kitson A and McKnight T (1992) *Challenges in Caring: Explorations in Nursing and Ethics.* London: Chapman and Hall.

Brown R (1965) *Social Psychology.* London: Collier Macmillan.

Candee D and Puka B (1988) An analytic approach to resolving problems in medical ethics. In J Dowie and A Elstein *Professional Judgment: A Reader in Clinical Decision Making.* Cambridge: Cambridge University Press, pp. 474–91.

Davis A and Aroskar M (1983) *Ethical Dilemmas and Nursing Practice* (2nd edn.). Norwalk, Conn.: Appleton Century Crofts.

Deaux K, Dane F and Wrightsman L (1993) *Social Psychology in the 90's* (6th edn.). Pacific Grove, CA: Brooks/Cole.

Festinger L (1964) The motivating effect of cognitive dissonance. In R Harper, C Anderson, C Christensen and S Hunka *The Cognitive Processes: Readings.* Englewood Cliffs, NJ: Prentice Hall, pp. 509–23.

Greipp M (1992) Greipp's model of ethical decision making. *Journal of Advanced Nursing,* 17: pp. 734–8.

Heckhausen H and Weiner B (1972) The emergence of a cognitive psychology of motivation. In P Dodwell *New Horizons in Psychology, 2.* Harmondsworth, Middlesex: Penguin Education, pp. 126–47.

Husted G and Husted J (1991) *Ethical Decision Making in Nursing.* St Louis, Miss: C V Mosby.

Johnson A (1990) *Pathways in Medical Ethics.* London: Edward Arnold.

Johnstone M (1989) *BioEthics: A Nursing Perspective.* London: Harcourt Brace Jovanovich.

Lippa R (1990) *Introduction to Social Psychology.* Belmont, Calif: Wadsworth.

Marquis B and Huston C (1992) *Leadership Roles and Management Functions in Nursing: Theory and Application.* Philadelphia: J B Lippincott.

Pellegrino E (1981) *A Philosophical Basis of Medical Practice:*

Toward a Philosophy and Ethic of the Healing Professions. New York: Oxford University Press.

Purtilo R (1993) *Ethical Dimensions in the Health Professions* (2nd edn.). Philadelphia, W B Saunders.

Radford J and Govier E (eds.) (1980) *A Textbook of Psychology.* London: Sheldon Press.

Rumbold G (1986) *Ethics in Nursing Practice.* London: Baillière Tindall.

Seedhouse D (1988) *Ethics: The Heart of Health Care.* Chichester: John Wiley and Sons.

Seedhouse D (1991) *Liberating Medicine.* Chichester: John Wiley and Sons.

Seedhouse D and Lovett L (1992) *Practical Medical Ethics.* Chichester: John Wiley and Sons.

Thompson I, Melia K and Boyd K (1988) *Nursing Ethics* (2nd edn.). London: Churchill Livingstone.

Tschudin V (1992) *Ethics in Nursing: The Caring Relationship* (2nd edn.). Oxford: Butterworth Heinemann.

UKCC (1992) *Code of Professional Conduct* (3rd edn.). London: UKCC.

Uustal D (1990) Enhancing your ethical reasoning. *Critical Care Nursing Clinics of North America*, 2 (3): pp. 437–42.

Index